Hospital Security Guard
Training Manual

Hospital Security Guard Training Manual

By

JOHN A. WANAT

Director
Cooperative Vocational Technical Education
New Jersey State Department of Education

JOHN F. BROWN

Safety and Security Director
St. Joseph's Hospital and Medical Center
Paterson, New Jersey

LAWRENCE C. CONNIN

Chief (Retired)
Fire Prevention Bureau
Jersey City Fire Department

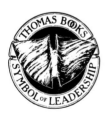

CHARLES   C   THOMAS   •   PUBLISHER
Springfield • Illinois • U.S.A.

Published and Distributed Throughout the World by
CHARLES C THOMAS ● PUBLISHER
Bannerstone House
301-327 East Lawrence Avenue, Springfield, Illinois, U.S.A.

© *1977, by* CHARLES C THOMAS ● PUBLISHER
ISBN 0-398-03656-X
Library of Congress Catalog Card Number: 77-1390

With THOMAS BOOKS *careful attention is given to all details of
manufacturing and design. It is the Publisher's desire to present books that
are satisfactory as to their physical qualities and artistic possibilities and
appropriate for their particular use.* THOMAS BOOKS *will be true to those
laws of quality that assure a good name and good will.*

Printed in the United States of America
R-1

Library of Congress Cataloging in Publication Data
Wanat, John A
  Hospital security guard training manual.

  Bibliography: p.
  Includes index.
  1. Hospitals--Security measures. I. Brown, John
Francis, 1932- joint author. II. Connin, Lawrence C.,
joint author. III. Title.
RA969.95.W36   363.2   77-1390
ISBN 0-398-03656-X

PREFACE

THE security officer of today's hospital must be able to deal with thefts, fires, accidents, bomb scares, distressed visitors, and safety hazards. The days of simply dressing a man in a guard's uniform to stand at the front door are gone. Today's security officer is a member of the third largest industry in the world — hospitals. This business's purchases total billions of dollars a year and, as all big businesses are aware, the losses associated with thefts are staggering. But theft *control* is only one facet of a hospital security officer's duties. He must also be able to identify potential safety hazards, confine and extinguish fires, and coordinate disaster control plans.

The complex task of a hospital security officer demands proper training so that he can effectively and efficiently carry out his assignments. For this reason, this text is addressed to the hospital security officer. Its purpose is to provide basic information and instructions relative to the performance of duties. It is designed as a general guide, a ready reference manual, to assist on the job. The subject content should appeal to the new hospital security officer, but the experienced officer will also find, in the selection of material, those references which he most frequently has occasion to consult. Each hospital is unique in its own physical layout, size, population, and problems; therefore, some techniques listed in this text will have to be modified individually to suit each particular situation while other techniques are basic and germane to all hospital security operations.

This text is divided into three major parts: the organization and development of a professional hospital security force, chapters 1 through 5; security operations and controls, chapters 6 through 17; and hospital safety as it relates to fires, bombs, and hazards, chapters 8 through 22. In addition, accompanying each chapter are handy reference lists that supplement the subject areas.

Chapters 21 and 22 are adopted from All About OSHA, pamphlet OSHA 2056, and Organizing a Safety Committee, pamphlet OSHA 2231, both issued by the United States Department of Labor, Occupational Safety and Health Administration. Indebtedness to these vital and thorough publications and the U. S. Department of Labor is gratefully acknowledged.

The authors are aware of the limited formal training, both in-service and public, and the lack of sufficient formal publications in this field. They are also aware of the field's desire to improve this situation. With this in mind, the authors endeavor to provide the field with a functional manual that will cover the important aspects of establishing and maintaining a strong workable security force. It is our hope that it will provide the necessary elements to spur on more in-house training as well as formal training by outside educational training institutions and agencies.

ACKNOWLEDGMENTS

THIS book is dedicated with deep appreciation to the wives, Arlene, Anita, and Lena; and children of the authors. We are especially grateful to the following organizations and institutions for their contributions to this text: Frontier Security Inc.; Jersey City State College, Center For Occupational Education: St. Joseph's Hospital and Medical Center; ADT Security Systems; Visual Methods Incorporated; St. Barnabas Medical Center; Rutgers University Curriculum Laboratory; The Center For Career and Vocational Education, Western Kentucky University; International Association for Hospital Security; National Institute for Occupational Safety and Health; Holy Name Hospital; Muhlenburg Hospital; The American Hospital Association and The National Safety Council.

Finally, we express our sincere gratitude to all those who have assisted us with their advice and efforts in preparing this text; and a special thanks to Arlene Wanat, Alfreda Obornik, and Margaret Austin for their typing and productive clerical suggestions.

CONTENTS

Section III. Hospital Safety

Hospital Security Guard
Training Manual

Section I

Organization and Development

Chapter 1

WHY HOSPITALS NEED SECURITY

TODAY'S modern hospital is analogous to today's modern drug store. Both are more than their names imply. Although both facilities are dedicated to the care and treatment of patient's ills, they have expanded in size and scope to be more than they were a decade ago.

The hospitals of today are modern, complex facilities often consisting of numerous physical buildings, encompassing entire city blocks, and housing hundreds and even thousands of patients, professional staff, and supportive personnel — not to mention the countless numbers of visitors, distributors, and service personnel who enter and exit the hospital each day. In this vast, modern, complex structure known as a hospital, the protection of patients, employees, visitors, and property has an ever greater meaning for hospital administrators. It is no longer acceptable, nor feasible, to ignore the importance of a professional security force in today's hospital.

The capital investment of all U. S. hospitals today is in excess of 30 billion dollars. It is the third largest industry, surpassing the investment in automobiles, railroads, and even telephone communications.

The responsibility of the hospital administrator is a formidable one, indeed. The operation of a hospital is not only big business, but a complex of many big businesses. The administration must contend with the problems of building maintenance; a pharmacy, hotel, laundry, restaurant, purchasing department, research and educational institution. (Norman Jaspan: Structuring Security in a Hospital. *Empire State Architect.*)

This type of complex business makes security control a difficult task. It becomes an impossible task when hospital administrators ignore the development of a well-rounded security operation. A conscientious effort with full administrative

5

backing is needed for security personnel to develop a workable security system within a hospital. That system should be able to accomplish the following:

(1) PROTECTION OF LIFE AND PROPERTY. This can be achieved by periodic tours of the hospital and grounds, by providing escort service for personnel during late evening hours, and by the establishment of twenty-four-hour-a-day guard coverage, especially in the Emergency Service area.

(2) PRESERVATION OF THE PEACE. This would include the restraint and/or removal of disorderly persons from the hospital. Quite often, problems develop in the treatment of alcoholics, drug addicts, and psychiatric patients.

(3) PREVENTION OF VANDALISM AND OTHER CRIMES. This is the result of good patrolling, which results in a considerable savings to the hospital.

(4) PREVENTION AND DETECTION OF FIRE AND SAFETY HAZARDS. Included in this responsibility are watch clock tours — fire checks during the late evening hours. Security personnel while touring the hospital should also take the opportunity to note and report obvious safety hazards.

(5) ENFORCEMENT OF HOSPITAL RULES AND REGULATIONS. This includes such items as visitor pass control, enforcement of parking regulations and fire and safety codes, and the enforcement of hospital policies in general.

A security program can have many different applications depending on the size of the hospital and its individual needs. In addition to the basic responsibilities previously outlined, security services can be geared to include investigations of accidents or incidents on hospital property, maintaining a lost and found department, traffic control, issuance of parking decals, issuance of personnel identification cards, and similar duties.

No two security programs are identical. There is, however, a body of general knowledge, rules, and regulations common to all efficient security programs. Given the basics essential to all hospital security programs, and depending on the physical layout, type and size of the hospital, and environmental aspects, security should be programmed to fit individual hospital needs.

The security program serves many purposes. It fulfills the

hospital's obligation to protect the premises against fire and safety hazards as well as against persons who would do harm to patients, visitors, and employees. In addition, security service provides a physical and psychological barrier to deter antisocial behavior.

Unfortunately, we live in a society where antisocial behavior is very much a part of the scene, where drug abuse has reached an all time high, and where alcoholics and mental patients line the emergency wards and often fill our hospitals to capacity.

The question is not "Why do hospitals need security?" Rather the real question is "How can hospitals afford being without it?"

SELECTED READINGS

Ann, Sister Patricia: Why we leave our security program to professionals, *Hospitals,* January 1960.

Brownfield, H.: Hospital security. *Michigan Hospital,* 5:August 1969.

Burns, D. Bruce: *National Survey on Hospital Security.* Briarcliff Manor, New York: Burns Security Institute, October 1972.

Chaden, Sydney: Security is a condition. *Security World,* 5(3):23-26, March 1968.

Cole, R. B.: Designing for security. *Progressive Architect,* 51:84-89, November 1970.

Collins, Russel: Hospital: What it means and how to achieve it. *Hospitals,* 41:67-69, November 16, 1967.

Daley, Robert W.: Security important in hospitals. *Safety Newsletter:* National Safety Council, August 1970, p. 1.

Gilmer, Sam O., Jr.: How should the administrator organize a security program? *Modern Hospital, 103,* No. 1:83-85, July 1964.

How hospitals buy security by contract. *Modern Hospital, 103,* No. 1:86-89, July 1964.

Linn, William C.: For you, what is "Security"? *Hospital Management, 102,* No. 3:70-74, September 1966.

McShea, Kevin Michael: *Expansion of the Present Concept of Hospital Security: A Managerial Perspective.* International Association for Hospital Security.

Marcus, Stanley: Management looks at security. *Industrial Security,* October 1960.

Schnalbolk, Charles: Sensible security for an irrational decade. *Buildings,* 64:52-55, July 1970.

Chapter 2

ORGANIZATION

Organization

THE organization of a good hospital security officer (guard) force is dependent upon a cooperative, well organized, military style line and staff structure. The supervisory channels and operations are as follows:

(1) SECURITY DIRECTOR. Hospital security guards are generally under the direction and supervision of a security director. As an administrator, he reports to an assistant administrator of the hospital or directly to the director of the hospital. The security director is responsible for the overall security operations of the hospital. The security director plans, develops, and administers hospital protection programs, including security guard training programs. He also provides professional security advice to hospital officials and maintains a close liaison with the local fire and law enforcement agencies.

(2) ASSISTANT SECURITY DIRECTOR. In hospitals of significant size, the director of security has an assistant who coordinates with the director in planning and implementation of security operations. He carries out the orders and directions of the director and, in his absence, acts for the director.

(3) ORGANIZATIONAL CHART. In order to clearly define levels of responsibility and authority, it is recommended that an organizational survey first be taken and then an organizational chart be developed. Once developed and implemented, any changes in the organization must be approved by the hospital director. Figure 1 is an illustration chart which shows the line of authority.

(4) HOSPITAL SECURITY GUARD QUALIFICATIONS. At the present time, there are no formal set standards for hospital security guards, and requirements will vary from hospital to hospital. There are, however, desirable attributes that each

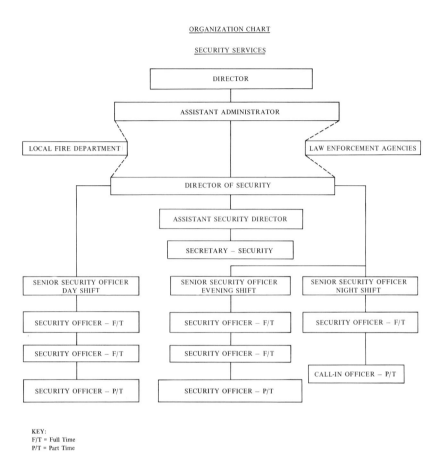

ORGANIZATION CHART

SECURITY SERVICES

DIRECTOR

ASSISTANT ADMINISTRATOR

LOCAL FIRE DEPARTMENT

LAW ENFORCEMENT AGENCIES

DIRECTOR OF SECURITY

ASSISTANT SECURITY DIRECTOR

SECRETARY – SECURITY

SENIOR SECURITY OFFICER DAY SHIFT

SENIOR SECURITY OFFICER EVENING SHIFT

SENIOR SECURITY OFFICER NIGHT SHIFT

SECURITY OFFICER – F/T

SECURITY OFFICER – F/T

SECURITY OFFICER – F/T

SECURITY OFFICER – F/T

SECURITY OFFICER – F/T

CALL-IN OFFICER – P/T

SECURITY OFFICER – P/T

SECURITY OFFICER – P/T

KEY:
F/T = Full Time
P/T = Part Time

Figure 1.

security director should look for when considering applicants for a guard's position:

(a) Physical fitness to carry out assignments and responsibilities.
(b) Ability to communicate verbally and in writing.
(c) Ability to learn and enforce rules and guidelines.
(d) Ability to take orders and give them.
(e) Ability to deal with people.
(f) Tact and courtesy.

(g) Loyalty, integrity, and honesty.

(h) Alertness.

(i) Conscientiousness.

(j) Ability to demonstrate good judgment.

(k) Ability to be firm in applying protection procedures, methods, and techniques.

(5) THE OFFICERS' FUNCTIONS. Hospital security guards are full or part-time, institutional or contract; they are uniformed employees assigned to protect the hospital's patients, visitors, employees, equipment, and physical facilities against the hazards of theft, fire, safety, damage, accidents, trespass, sabotage, and bombs. They must maintain positive prevention and enforce the hospital's regulations.

(6) RANK OF OFFICERS. The size, operations, and organizational chart of a hospital will determine the need for the officer ranks that a hospital employs. A fully staffed guard organization is composed of captain(s), lieutenant(s), sergeant(s), and private(s) in sufficient numbers to provide reasonable guard protection under adequate supervision. When a hospital does not require full staffing in all ranks, supervisory channels may be changed or adjusted. The overall protection duties and responsibilities, however, remain the same. The basic duties and responsibilities set forth below are typical of hospital guard operations in each rank.

(a) *Captain.* A security captain is the highest ranking officer assigned to an assistant or chief security director. The captain generally serves as the officer in charge of one of the tours of duty, with the direct supervision of security lieutenant(s) and security sergeant(s) and overall supervision of the officers (guards) on his relief. He carries out the orders and instructions of the security director or assistant director. In the absence of the chief security director and/or his assistant, he acts for the director. He assigns guards to their tour, makes daily inspections, trains lieutenants to act in his place during his absence, advises the director of unusual happenings, acts as a rating officer for subordinates, and remains within his area of responsibility until properly relieved, advising headquarters of his whereabouts at all times while on duty.

(b) *Lieutenant.* When a lieutenant is the highest ranking officer, his duties and responsibilities are the same as those of a captain. When under the supervision of a captain, the lieutenant generally serves as the officer in charge of one of the reliefs of duty, with the direct supervision of security sergeants and overall supervision of the guards on his relief. He carries out the orders and instructions of the captain and, in his absence, acts for the captain. He assigns guards on his relief, makes daily inspections, trains sergeants to act in his place during his absence, advises the captain of unusual happenings, acts as rating officer for subordinates, and remains within his area of responsibility until properly relieved, advising headquarters of his whereabouts at all times while on duty.

(c) *Sergeant.* When the highest ranking officer assigned to the hospital, his duties and responsibilities are the same as a captain or lieutenant, as the situation indicates. When under the supervision of a lieutenant, he exercises direct supervision over guard privates within his area. He carries out the orders and instructions of the lieutenant, and, in his absence, assumes his authority and responsibilities. He makes guard and building inspections, advises his superior of guard activities and unusual events, trains guards to act for him in his absence, evaluates the performance of guards under his jurisdiction, and maintains contact with headquarters, remaining within his area of responsibility until properly relieved.

(d) *Guard.* A security guard is under the immediate supervision of a sergeant. His job is to protect the building or buildings and grounds to which he is assigned, including the contents, occupants, and visitors and make patrols as assigned. He seeks out and takes immediate protective action against existing hazards or conditions which may cause damage, injury, or interference through fire, accident, theft, or trespass and reports such conditions or hazards by use of established hospital security forms (see chapter 17). He enforces security regulations where applicable, handles lost and found articles, enforces rules and regulations governing the building, and directs traffic. He uses special police authority when it is vested in him to make arrests for cause or, when no such authority exists, calls upon available law enforcement personnel to make necessary arrests. He maintains order on his post and helps persons requiring assistance or information, observes good guarding practices and standards, and performs such other duties as are assigned.

Suggested Hospital Security Guard Employment Practices and Work Requirements

EMPLOYEE INFORMATION. Every new employee should receive information on how pay is determined, health and safety requirements, training opportunities, conduct regulations, and work related or fringe benefits information.

WORK REQUIREMENTS. A hospital security guard is part of an organizational structure that requires all concerned to operate in an effective and orderly manner.

(a) *Schedule.* A work schedule for a predetermined time is posted and distributed to all concerned.

(b) *Key Posts.* Some guard posts cannot be left unmanned at any point in time. Those assigned to such a post will remain there until properly relieved. These posts will be distinctly spelled out in the hospital's rules and regulations.

(c) *Tour of Duty.* All hospital security guards will be in full uniform and at their respective posts on time and shall remain on the job and carry out their assignments until the end of their full tour of duty when they are properly relieved of duty.

(d) *Lunch Hours.* All guards are authorized a designated time for their lunch period. A security officer is on duty while at lunch and is subject to call.

GUARD IDENTIFICATION. Each guard should be issued an official identification card and badge to be carried on his person while on official duty. The identification should not be used for any purpose other than official hospital duty and if lost or

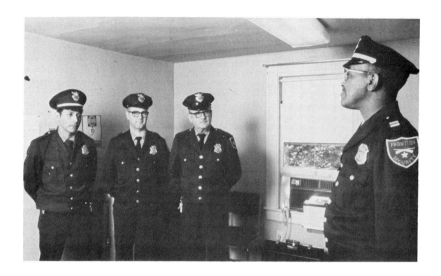

Figure 2. Security officers line up for daily inspection and post assignments. (*Courtesy of* Frontier Security, Inc.)

stolen, an official report should be made out immediately.

RESIDENCE AND TELEPHONE REGISTRATION. Each guard should have on permanent file in the security office his home address and telephone number. Any change in residence or phone number should be immediately corrected. His file should also include any language(s) he speaks fluently.

CONDUCT ON THE JOB. Each guard is expected to carry out his assignments in the highest ethical manner. He must observe the strictest requirements of courtesy, consideration, and promptness in dealing with patients, visitors, staff, superiors, and local fire and police authorities.

(a) *Hospital telephone usage.* Personal calls are not to be made on hospital phones at any time. All incoming calls should be answered in a pleasant, businesslike manner with the officer stating his location, name, and rank. Assistance should be of prime importance.

(b) *Sleeping on duty.* Sleeping on duty is strictly forbidden and subject to disciplinary action and/or dismissal. The protection of visitors, patients, and staff is dependent upon his alertness and quick response to a given situation.

(c) *Foul language.* A guard should not engage in the use of foul language while on the job. It takes away from his professional image and should not be tolerated.

(d) *Private reading, talking, and listening to a private radio or television* while on duty are not permitted. A guard cannot carry out his duties with undivided attention if he is so engaged.

(e) *Drinking and narcotics* are strictly forbidden on the job.

(f) *Smoking and chewing gum* while on duty should be limited and reserved for breaks.

SELECTED READINGS

Davis, James A.: What is a security director? *Industrial Security,* December 1970.

GSA Handbook, Physical Protection (PBSP5930.2A) Organization General Service Administration, Washington, D.C., Chapter 9, part 2, September 1970.

Healy, Richard J.: Putting security on the management team. *Security World,* 2, No. 5:July-August 1965.

International Association For Hospital Security: Security standards for large institutions. *Security World,* December 1971.

Jupiter, Robert M.: Hospital security plan should coordinate with city plan. *Modern Hospital, 110:*72, 76, 80, June 1968.

Momboisse, Raymond M.: *Industrial Security For Strikes, Riots and Disasters.* Springfield, Thomas, 1972.

Post, Richard S. and Kingsbury, Arthur A.: *Security Administration, An Introduction,* 2nd Ed. Springfield, Thomas, 1973.

Staffing for security. *Canadian Security Gazette,* October 1971.

Chapter 3

PROFESSIONAL APPEARANCE
AND CHARACTERISTICS

A HOSPITAL security guard should maintain the highest standards of personal appearance. Good grooming and careful attention to one's uniform are a *must* for the security officer who wishes to command respect from those he serves. A security guard's uniform is a symbol of authority and respect. However, the uniform itself does not make others respect the man or the position he holds. The man must do that himself.

   (a) A security officer should wear uniforms that are in good repair. There should be no missing buttons, no frayed collars and cuffs, and no ripped seams.
   (b) His uniform should be clean and pressed. His uniform should not be soiled with grease spots, no baggy knees or elbows, and no dirty shoes.

A security officer is usually the first person one sees as he enters the hospital. If he looks sloppy, the visitor's first impression of the security force is poor and the confidence level is marred.

POSTURE. Good posture is important to the overall good appearance of the security guard. He should not slouch nor look awkward in his appearance. Good posture gives those who come in contact with the security guard the impression that he is in command and that he has confidence in himself and in his work.

PERSONALITY. A security guard should display courtesy, understanding, authority, honesty, and confidence. Everything he does while on the job should lead others to trust and respect him. When he is enforcing the hospital's rules on the number of visitors allowed in a room, he should be diplomatic and understanding. He still has a job to do, but the manner in which he speaks and acts will determine how effective a job he

15

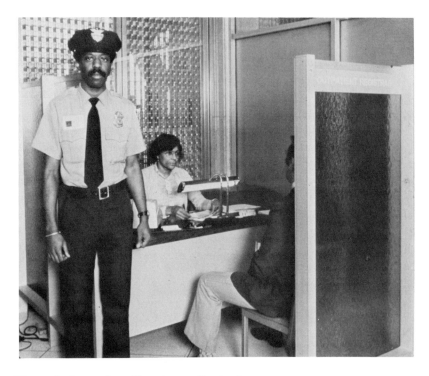

Figure 3. A security officer is usually the first person one sees when entering the hospital. If the security officer looks like a professional, he will usually be treated as one. (*Courtesy of* Frontier Security, Inc.)

is doing and the *good will* or *bad will* he creates with the visitor. More often than not, if the security officer's approach and tact are proper, he will succeed in carrying out his assignment without antagonizing the friends and family of a patient.

A security guard must always be patient and courteous with visitors, patients, hospital personnel, and all others he comes in contact with. It is not always easy to be patient and courteous, but he must remember patients and visitors are under emotional strain and are not always themselves.

A security guard must always be tactful when approaching anyone. He should never give anyone the opportunity to complain.

Above all else, a security guard has a responsibility to carry out the hospital's rules and regulations. He must, however, carry out these responsibilities in the highest professional manner. If someone enters the hospital and passes the information desk and guard, it is the guard's duty to approach the person in a polite manner and ask him where he is going. If the person is uncooperative and does not have proper identification, the guard should try to prevent him from proceeding any further by stepping in front of him. The guard should again ask the person to state his business at the hospital, while making the person aware of the hospital's rules and regulations. If the person still refuses to cooperate, then it is the guard's duty to call his immediate superior and the local police. If the guard is handling the situation correctly, the person is trespassing and the guard is performing his duty by signing the complaint. It is then the responsibility of the police to remove the person from the property.

APPENDIX

Security Officer Inspection Checklist

SECURITY OFFICER_____ POST # _____

Knowledge of Duties   *Personal Appearance*

Excellent ( ) Satisfactory   ( )   Excellent ( ) Satisfactory   ( )

Good   ( ) Unsatisfactory ( )   Good   ( ) Unsatisfactory ( )

Post Appearance   *Attitude*

Excellent ( ) Satisfactory   ( )   Excellent ( ) Satisfactory   ( )

Good   ( ) Unsatisfactory ( )   Good   ( ) Unsatisfactory ( )

_____

ADDITIONAL REMARKS:

_____

INSTRUCTIONS:

This report is to be completed by supervisor on duty at time of inspection.

_____

Signature of Authorized Supervisor   Date   Time

_____

Courtesy of St. Joseph's Hospital and Medical Center, Paterson, New Jersey.

SELECTED READINGS

Coultier, Richard L.: Goodby guard, hello Joe. *Industrial Security,* October 1971.

Foster, Willard O., Jr.: The invisible alcoholic. *Industrial Security,* 2:9, December 1967.

Goddard, Robert J.: Professionalism in security — Fact or fiction. *Industrial Security, 9*:10, January 1965.

GSA Handbook Physical Protection (PBSP5930.2A) Chapter 9, part 4, Employment Practices and Requirements, General Service Administration, Washington, D.C., September 1970.

Potter, Anthony N., Jr.: Uniforms and security. *Industrial Security,* October 1970.

Scholl, C. E., Dr.: Professionalism and ... you. *Industrial Security, 9*:10, January 1965.

Security Guidelines For Hospitals, The Greater New York Hospital Association, New York, 1968.

Security officer — Newly emerging specialist in modern hospital's preventive medicine. *The Cornett* (St. Joseph Hospital, Chicago) 7, No. 8: August 1969. (Appears in Colling, Russell L., Ed.: *Hospital Security and Safety Journal Articles.* New York, Med Exam, 1970, pp. 26-27.)

Wathen, Thomas W.: *Security Subjects: An Officer's Guide to Plant Protection.* Springfield, Thomas, 1972.

Chapter 4

HUMAN RELATIONS*

HUMAN relations may be defined as one's ability to interact favorably with others. It may further take on an additional meaning, namely, that others are able to favorably accept us and thus favorably interact with us. Human relations, then, is favorable interpersonal and intergroup relations.

An underlying concept of human relations is the understanding of, and the sensitivity to, individual differences. It is not sufficient to understand individual differences, we must be able to accept individual differences. Under normal conditions, positive human relations is often a difficult task. The degree of difficulty becomes greater when we have to maintain effective human relations under stress conditions. The security officer is constantly facing stress conditions within a hospital setting. The best means to maintain positive human relations, under any given set of circumstances, is to display positive behavior and positive attitude at all times.

The authors have chosen not to elaborate on individual differences as they relate to race, creed, color, religion, social or economic status, political affiliations etc. Numerous texts are devoted to this phase of the subject area. The authors have, therefore, decided to approach this subject by concentrating on desirable personality traits of a hospital security officer. If we can understand how our personality traits and our working relations affect ourselves and others, then we will have a better understanding of the human relation's concept.

To begin, personality traits are intangible and are not easy to explain or understand. Nevertheless, it is essential that each individual understands the meaning and importance of the

---

*Portions of this chapter were adopted with permission of Dr. Clayton Riley from *Human Relations,* Bowling Green, Center For Career and Vocational Education, Western Kentucky University, June 1974, pp. 50-71.

proper use of these traits, and their relationship to success on the job. People can acquire these traits or improve their use of them, if they are willing to put forth effort. An officer with a good personality will treat people as individuals, not pass the buck, be loyal, go about the job cheerfully, help others when they need help, seek promotion on the basis of merit, and be honest, patient, and sincere.

A pleasing personality can assist the security officer in succeeding by understanding several points. First, a personality is comprised of the traits and characteristics — physical, mental, and emotional — that make up a whole person. Such traits include friendliness, helpfulness, tactfulness, enthusiasm, initiative, industry, dependability, and interest in others. Second, self-control is a very important trait. Self-control contributes to poise and patience. There is no place in the security field for an individual who does not have self-control. Third, the way a person speaks reveals his personality as much as the rest of his appearance. Regardless of how well-dressed a person may be, crudities of speech can betray him. Although speech is not an indication of character, a good voice conveying good English is a convincing factor. Tone, pitch, rate, volume, and quality of one's voice can be improved. Enunciation and pronunciation are important. One must be aware of needed improvement before he can initiate actions to correct his deficiencies. The use of improper terms and curse words is a sure indication of poor manners, lack of self-control, and a limited vocabulary.

Fourth, self-improvement can occur if one knows what needs improving and develops a plan of action. A suggested plan for personality self-improvement is as follows:

a. Decide to improve.
b. Take an initial inventory of habits, attitudes, and traits.
c. Imitate a desired personality, keeping the image constantly in mind.
d. Work on one habit or trait at a time until it is acceptable, then proceed to another trait.
e. Substitute good habits for poor habits and practice the good habit constantly, using the help of friends and suggestions from all sources.

   f. Make periodic progress checks and adjust the improvement plan as necessary.

A Self-inventory of Desirable Characteristics

Listed below are sixty desirable characteristics. No one person will demonstrate all of these characteristics, but, a person with a desirable personality will demonstrate an abundance of them, while striving to incorporate all of them.

Desirable Characteristics	*Always*	*Most of the Time*	*Sometimes*	*Occasionally*	*Never*
1. Conscientiousness					
2. Neatness of Appearance					
3. Good Grooming					
4. Good Hygiene					
5. Energy					
6. Ambition					
7. Honesty					
8. Self-Awareness					
9. Consideration					
10. Friendliness					
11. Understanding Nature					
12. Extroversion					
13. Sociability					
14. Dependability					
15. Alertness					
16. Loyalty					
17. Good Citizenship					
18. Good Judgment					
19. Industriousness					
20. Leadership Qualities					
21. Ability to be Liked by Others					
22. Cooperativeness					
23. Ability to Take Correction Graciously					
24. Ability to Plan Well					
25. Cheerfulness					
26. Good Speech Habits					
27. Calmness Under Stress					
28. Self-Control					
29. Tactfulness					
30. Respect for Property of Others					

Desirable Characteristics	Always	Most of the Time	Sometimes	Occasionally	Never
31. Creativity					
32. Charitability					
33. Team Spirit					
34. High Ideals					
35. Humility					
36. Ability to Learn by Mistakes					
37. Ability to Gain by Experiences					
38. Promptness					
39. Courteousness					
40. Thriftiness					
41. Purposefulness					
42. Patience					
43. Positive Attitude					
44. Adaptability					
45. Maturity					
46. Emotional Stability					
47. Trustworthiness					
48. Ability to be a Good Loser					
49. Striving for Self-Improvement					
50. Intellectual Curiosity					
51. Conversational Ability					
52. Sincerity					
53. Poise					
54. Good Manners					
55. Sympathetic Demeanor					
56. Efficiency					
57. Good Memory					
58. Imagination					
59. Persistence					
60. Sense of Humor					

HOW OUR WORKING RELATIONS AFFECT
OURSELVES AND OTHERS

Our attitudes and behavior affect those around us because interaction between persons is constant. Our conduct can make others more or less efficient, thus doing our best helps in the overall efficiency of the hospital. Adapting easily to job and hospital regulations smoothes away friction; troublemakers and complainers do not keep jobs long.

A positive attitude is important for several reasons. Attitude is more than a smile or frown, since they reflect attitudes. We reveal our attitudes by what we see or look for in a job or supervisor, how we deal with our associates, and our desire to be of service to others. Concentration on the positive, constructive, helpful aspects of a job breeds energy and initiative. Every job has some unpleasant or negative features, but concentration on what we dislike drains away energy and enthusiasm.

Tension and anger can be discharged constructively. We must realize that no human relationships are always smooth; pentup anger is a common problem in security. We must also recognize that tension and anger may arise over situations we cannot change. Work out your depression, anxiety, and restlessness in some positive and vigorous activity: a brisk, long walk, or swimming for example. Talk out frustration in private with a person you trust.

Why People Fail As Employees

Harvard University interviewed 4,375 graduates who had failed as employees. Results of the survey revealed that 34.2 percent failed because of lack of technical knowledge, while 65.8 percent were discharged because of a lack of personality development and adjustment.

Thirteen Reasons Why Most People Fail

(1) Unwillingness to cooperate with or help others.
(2) Discourteousness, rudeness, and indifference to the other

fellow's interests, wants, desires, and point of view.
(3) Unreliability, lack of dependability.
(4) Carelessness, indifference, the "so what" attitude: "I'll get by."
(5) "Cutting the other fellow down to size," too free with the stinging rebuke and the humiliating remark, making fun of others.
(6) Desire to domineer, wanting to boss others, acting superior.
(7) Troublemaking, agitating, being always dissatisfied, the-world-owes-me-a-living attitude.
(8) Laziness, loafing on the job, habitual lateness.
(9) Disagreeableness, lack of respect for others, the "I'm-right-but-the-world's-all-wrong attitude."
(10) Misconduct, violation of rules, unwillingness to conform to prescribed standards recognized as essential for the well-being of all.
(11) Drinking to excess.
(12) Dishonesty.
(13) Absenteeism, found wanting in the sense of responsibility.

Undesirable Security Officer Traits That Can Destroy Human Relations Within a Hospital

Being impolite to visitors.
Being unfriendly with hospital staff.
Being jealous.
Using foul language.
Loafing on the job.
Displaying unsatisfactory attitudes.
Displaying lack of interest or concern.
Displaying lack of initiative.
Being irresponsible.
Assuming more authority than authorized.
Degrading other people.
Being indifferent to suggestions and criticisms.
Griping constantly.
Gossiping about everyone.

Demonstrating lack of self control.
Exploiting other people.

The Following Should Become the Security Officers Human Relation's Creed

- I am calm and patient under trying conditions.
- I am careful not to become hostile and sarcastic.
- I talk in a friendly, quiet tone of voice.
- I do not hold grudges against people.
- I am careful not to make gestures or grimaces.
- I am tolerant of other people's ideas and customs.
- I control my desire to make wisecracks.
- I am careful not to gossip.
- I am careful not to make fun of anyone.

SELECTED READINGS

Cosentino, Salvatore: *Public Relations and The Hospital Security Officer*, a paper presented at The Fifth Annual Institute for Hospital Security Guards, Greater New York Hospital Association, 1971.

Davis, Keith: *Human Relations At Work*. New York, McGraw, 1962.

Holcomb, Richard L.: *The Police and the Public*. Springfield, Thomas, 1975.

The Police Administration and Public Safety College of Social Science, Michigan State University: *Law and Order Training for Civil Defense Emergency, Student Manual* (Part B). East Lansing, Mich St U Pr, August 1965.

Neeson, John V.: Public relations and security. *Security World*, 3(9):15, October 1966.

Role of The Security Department In Human and Community Relations. *Security Education Briefs* (OAK Security Inc.), Vol. 2, No. 12.

Wathen, Thomas W.: *Security Subjects: An Officer's Guide to Plant Protection*. Springfield, Thomas, 1972.

Chapter 5

HOSPITAL SECURITY OFFICER TRAINING — A PROPOSED MODEL

THE authors, having been deeply involved in the developmental stages of what is now considered a very successful training program, offer a brief historical overview of the hospital security training program at Jersey City State College, Jersey City, New Jersey. In addition, the authors propose that the Jersey City State College Hospital Security Training program be considered a model for adoption by other colleges, agencies, and security organizations in developing a recognized formal training program for hospital security personnel.

"Education and training is becoming more important in security work and hospital security departments are beginning to realize the importance of formalized training programs." The statement is taken from a "flyer" by staff members of the Center For Occupational Education at Jersey City State College, Jersey City, New Jersey. The purpose of the flyer was to encourage hospital administrators and security directors to provide their security officers with sufficient training to carry out their assignments in a professional manner.

National reports, such as the Rand Corporation report "The Private Police Industry: Its Nature and Extent, 1972," have indicated that "There is an admitted, as well as an apparent, lack of training for private security personnel" (Kakalik and Wildhorn, 1972). The day of the untrained and unqualified security guard is past. Our modern technical society demands that security forces be professionals and that they be trained to deal with the everchanging security environment.

The Rand Corporation Report states: "Typically guard recruits are inexperienced in security work, thus they generally have no previous training for the job. Only a few firms, generally those employing a relatively well-paid in-house guard force, require a prospective guard to have had prior quality security experience" (Kakalik and Wildhorn, 1972, p. 86). Additionally, up until now, there have been no set standards for uniform training on any national level.

The hospital security program at Jersey City State College provides a uniform curriculum for interested hospital security personnel in New Jersey. The Center For Occupational Education at Jersey City State College began offering a twenty-hour training program in February 1973 at the request of the Margaret Hauge/Pollack Hospitals in Jersey City. The request came to the college after a year or more of fruitless searching for an agency that would consider training the hospitals' private security guards. The college undertook a survey to determine the specific job functions of a hospital security officer. From this survey, they initiated the following ten-week, twenty-hour training program:

Week	*Content and Scope*	*Hours*
1. Fire Prevention and Inspection		2

    a. Orientation
    b. Procedures
    c. Corrective action
    d. Equipment maintenance

2. Fire Evacuation and Extinguishment		2

    a. Fire drill procedures
    b. Equipment usage
    c. Coordination between local police-fire and hospital personnel
    d. Preventive maintenance-public information

3. Law of Arrest — Search and Seizure		2

    a. Legal restrictions
    b. Citizens arrest
    c. Inspecting packages, etc.
    d. Guard-police relationship

4. Patrol Functions		2

    a. Security

   b. Preventive maintenance
   c. Safety
   d. Assistance

5. Public Relations — Education   2

   a. Internal — with the hospital staff, patients, and visitors
   b. Informing the public of fire regulations, etc.
   c. Sensitivity
   d. Psychology of handling people

6. Preventive Security   2

   a. Developing and maintaining a strong security system
   b. Developing spot checks for pilferage from hospital
   c. Effective use of name tags
   d. Controlling keys
   e. Fingerprinting new employees

7. Reports   2

   a. Types of reports
   b. Need for reports

8. Report Writing   2

   a. Contents
   b. Developing reports

9. Bomb Procedures   2

   a. Bomb threats
   b. Search
   c. Evacuation
   d. Cooperation internal-external
   e. What to look for

10. Safety   2

   a. Inspection tours
   b. Preventive measures
   c. Reports
   d. Corrective action
   e. Follow up
   f. Educating staff and public

In the spring of 1974, the International Association for Hospital Security endorsed the Jersey City State College Program. As a result of their combined efforts, a "Forty-Hour Hospital

Security Program" was initiated at the College. The program, designed to allow for mobility and transfer recognition throughout the country for a security officer having completed a standard Hospital Security Program, is outlined below:

Week	*Topic*	*Hours*
1.	Fire Prevention	2
2.	Fire Control	2
3.	Report and Report Writing	3
4.	Patrol Functions	3
5.	Organization	
	a. Security as a service organization	1
	b. Hospital organization	1
6.	Relations	
	a. Public	1/2
	b. Community	1/2
	c. Labor	1
7.	Laws of Arrest/Search/Seizure	2
8.	Hospital Safety	2
9.	Investigation/Interviews	2
10.	Narcotics and Dangerous Drugs	2
11.	Disaster Control	2
12.	Hospital Operations	
	a. Nursing	1
	b. Business office	1
	c. Ancillary services	1
	d. Food service	1
	e. Pharmacy	1
	f. Hospital vulnerabilities	1
13.	Bomb Procedures	2
14.	Physical Security Controls	1
15.	Law Enforcement Liaison	1
16.	Alarms	1
17.	Lock and Keys	1
18.	Equipment Usage/Maintenance	1
19.	Courtroom Procedures	1
20.	Disturbances	
	a. Civil	1
	b. Handling the patient, visitor, employee	1

The Hospital Security Program at Jersey City State College purpose is to provide in-service security personnel with a greater insight into their specific role in dealing with fires, thefts, assaults, disaster planning, and liability. The nature and responsibilities of the security officers are discussed and evaluated. In addition, the program is geared to assist security personnel in developing and implementing workable hospital security procedures.

The basic objectives of the JCSS-IAHS program are:

a. to establish minimum standards of basic training for the hospital security officer
b. to insure that training provided is of acceptable quality
c. to issue a recognized training certificate to each individual completing the basic requirements of the forty-hour program
d. to allow for mobility and transfer recognition throughout the country for a security officer having completed a standardized hospital security program.

The certificate program is offered on a dual track basis at various hospitals throughout the state, enabling security officers or other interested professionals to attend class on either one of two sessions. The same essential material is presented at both sessions by the same instructor. This dual teaching enables officers on rotating shifts to attend either one of the two sessions.

Qualified instructors are chosen for the program based upon their expertise in a specific area, along with high academic and practical experience. The security officer trainees, therefore, receive first hand information from professionals actively involved in the subject area they are presenting. Upon completion of the forty-hour program, a certificate of completion is issued to each participant by Jersey City State College. In addition, the International Association for Hospital Security, having endorsed the program, will issue full certification.

In summary, the authors strongly recommend that hospitals throughout the country adopt a formalized, standardized training program for their security officers. These programs should be flexible to adapt to changing needs and new technological advancements. The "forty-hour" training program presented on the preceding pages is not meant to be all-inclusive. Certainly, more hours can be devoted to each subject area. Unquestionably, there are other areas that can be included in the training package. If, however, all hospital security officers receive the common core outlined in the forty-hour program,

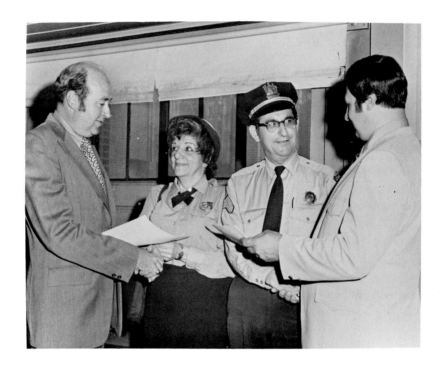

Figure 4. Security officers are awarded a certificate for satisfactorily completing a twenty-hour hospital security training program. (*Courtesy of* Jersey City State College.)

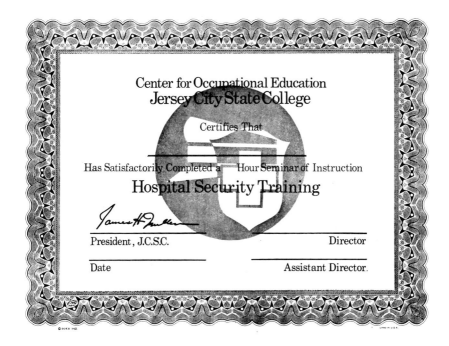

Center for Occupational Education
Jersey City State College

Certifies That

Has Satisfactorily Completed a ___ Hour Seminar of Instruction

Hospital Security Training

President, J.C.S.C.   Director

Date   Assistant Director.

Figure 5. (*Courtesy of* Jersey City State College.)

then security officers throughout the country would be that much closer in achieving their due professional recognition.

SELECTED READINGS

Astor, Saul D.: Operation audits to teach security. *Security World, 2* (No. 5):July-August 1965.

Badin, Fred P.: The security education program. *Industrial Security,* April 1968.

Caskey, C. C.: How to get more benefit from training. *Supervision,* October 1964.

Crowe, J. M.: Effective training reduces fire. *Industrial Security,* April 1960.

Curtis, S. J.: The psychology of security training. *Police,* May-June 1960.

Dangy, Gerald L.: Security education goals and principles. *Industrial Security,* December 1965.

Davis, Albert: "Towards Professionalism." *Industrial Security,* January 1968.

Dennis, Robert L.: Report of the ASIS education committee. *Industrial Security,* October 1963.

DeSanto, John F.: The key man. *Training Directors Manual,* July 19, 1965.

Despard, A.: *Management Review, 59*:60, February 1970.

Doherty, Joseph F. and Eugene B. Kelly: Seven steps to better security. *Industrial Security,* April 1962.

Elkins, E. V. and Reeder, J. A.: The answer to security training. *Industrial Security, 3* (No. 6): October 1959.

Formula to maximize security awareness. *Industrial Relations News, 13* (No. 22):June 1, 1963.

Germann, A. C.: Scientific training for industrial security. *Industrial Security,* January 1961.

Goddard, Robert J.: Security education and enforcement. *Industrial Security,* July 1961.

Hall, Wayne L.: Educator's challenge. *Industrial Security,* October 1961.

Handy, Jamison: The evolution of ideas, part 1. *Industrial Security.*

Hazelton, Tom: Educator's challenge. *Industrial Security,* October 1961.

Here security keeps pace with growth. *Industrial Security,* January 1964.

How to make your management security conscious. *Industrial Security, 6* (No. 2).

Johnson, Clarence L.: The scientist, the engineer and security. *Industrial Security,* October 1958.

Kakalik, James and Wildhorn, Sorrel: *The Private Police Industry:* Its Nature and Extent, Volume II, R-870/DOJ, The Rand Corporation, Santa Monica, California, 1971. Supported by The National Institute of Law Enforcement and Criminal Justice, U. S. Department of Justice, Superintendent of Documents, U. S. Government Printing Office, Washington, D. C., January 1967.

Kendall, Charles F. and Surles, Lynn: Operation training. *Journal American Society For Training,* June 1960.

Klotter, John C.: *Techniques For Police Instructors.* Springfield, Thomas, 1974.

Lewis, Howard L.: *In-House Security Department.* Chicago, McGraw, 1973.

Peel, John Donald: *Fundamentals of Training For Security Officers.* Springfield, Thomas, 1975.

Peel, John Donald: *The Training, Licensing and Guidance of Private Security Officers.* Springfield, Thomas, 1973.

Shane, Creamer G.: Private Police in The United States: Findings and Recommendations, a review. *Security World, 10*(4):30-69, April 1973.

Survey of Security Instruction Time. *Security World, 9*(2):24-25, February 1972.

"The Training of a Security Guard." *National Safety News, 103*:46-49, January 1971.

Section II

Security Operations and Controls

Chapter 6

HOSPITAL THEFT

IT was stated in Chapter 1 that hospitals are often huge complexes consisting of a multitude of businesses. It becomes extremely easy, therefore, for theft by employees, visitors, and vendors to occur within the hospital.

According to Norman Jaspan, President of Norman Jaspan Associates, Inc. (a leading management engineering firm) and author of *The Thief In The White Collar* and *Mind Your Own Business*, the opportunities for theft, waste, collusion, and all imaginable forms of malpractice in this (more than 8 billion dollars a year) industry stagger the imagination. Theft in supplies, equipment, food, drugs, narcotics, and other expendable goods intended for patients has become commonplace.

Items Stolen From a Hospital	*Location*
1. Linen such as pillow cases, sheets, towels, blankets, bedspreads, and mattress covers.	1. Housekeeping carts, linen closets, store rooms, hospital laundry, and receiving docks.
2. Power and hand tools, piping, wiring, lumber, and a multitude of engineering supplies and equipment.	2. Tool cribs, boiler rooms, and outlying storage areas.
3. Food such as meat, poultry, eggs, milk, coffee, fresh and canned fruit and vegetables.	3. Dietary Department, kitchen, restaurant or cafeteria, storage areas, freezers and coolers on floor kitchens and receiving areas.
4. Medical supplies such as cotton swabs, bandages, gauze, disposable syringes, tongue depressors, alcohol, hypodermic needles.	4. Emergency rooms, nursing stations, supply cabinets and rooms, general stores, clinics.
5. Medical equipment such as surgical instruments, stethoscopes, laryngoscopes.	5. Emergency rooms, doctor's and nursing quarters, lockers, labs, clinics.
6. Nursery items such as disposable diapers, lotions, newborn promotional gift samples.	6. Nursery, store rooms, receiving docks, general store rooms.

37

7. Merchandise such as magazines, jewelry, toys, flowers, watches, clothing, furniture, television sets, silverware.

7. Gift shops, patient's rooms, employee lockers, store rooms, dietary department, parking lots.

8. Office supplies and equipment such as stationary, pens, file folders, typewriters, adding machines.

8. Admittance office, billing department, nursing stations, all service departments, and general office areas.

9. Housekeeping supplies such as mops, pails, cleaners, brooms.

9. Store rooms, closets, and push carts.

10. Patients' belongings such as watches, money, credit cards, jewelry, clothing, radios.

10. Patient's room, locker and night stand, emergency rooms.

11. Employees' belongings such as clothing, money, umbrellas, watches, jewelry.

11. Employee lockers and automobiles, (nurses leave pocketbooks at nursing stations, as do other clerical and professional workers in offices).

12. Pharmaceuticals and drugs, the types and quantity range in the thousands of varieties.

12. Pharmacy, narcotic cabinets at each nursing station, emergency room, clinics, general store rooms.

13. Other — cars, equipment and furniture, photographic supplies and audio-visual equipment, cash, unauthorized telephone calls, falsification of employee time.cards, etc.

13. Parking lots, laboratories, classrooms and conference rooms, administrative offices, the entire hospital complex.

Who Steals and Why

The assumption that all theft is caused by outside forces is a fallacy. Another major fallacy is that theft does not occur with "trusted employees." Again quoting Norman Jaspan, "The largest percentage of the $10 billion ripped off annually by dishonest employees is accounted for by 'trusted' personnel, whose opportunities are great, whose methods are less subject to scrutiny and who are often the last to be suspected."

A close look at crime reports reveal that it is the trusted vice president or president of a bank who manipulates cash reserves, embezzles millions, and gambles away the depositor's savings. He is in a position where the opportunities are great and whose methods are less subject to scrutiny.

Likewise a doctor, trusted and dedicated as he may be, is prone to help himself to disposable syringes, cotton swabs, bandages, drugs, and other items. Although he can afford to buy his own, these items are in the open, available, and loosely inventoried. Besides, he may rationalize that he is not stealing; he is entitled to them, everybody is doing it, nobody will miss them, "I need them back at the office." The reasons why a person steals are numerous.

Another example of those who could steal in a hospital is the chef of the dietary department who may steal quantities of meats. He could stuff frozen meats in plastic bags to be thrown out with the garbage. Under the cover of darkness, he could transfer the discarded plastic bags into his car.

Others within the same department could steal items such as silverware, cups, individualized packaged coffee and cream, boxes of cereals, mayonnaise, ketchup, and anything else found in this department. They could store their loot in their lockers and later transfer it to shopping bags and packages to be taken home with them at the end of their shift.

The list of those who steal in a hospital can include (but not be limited to) doctors, nurses, kitchen employees, housekeepers, supervisors, technicians, professional employees, patients, visitors, vendors, maintenance employees, and even security personnel.

Some of the reasons why people steal in a hospital follow. "Everybody else is doing it." "The hospital owes it to me." "Nobody will miss what I'm taking." "The hospital's rich and can afford it." "I need these items at home." "I can sell what I take for a profit." "This will compensate me for being treated unfairly." "It's available."

What Can Be Done to Curtail Theft Within a Hospital

The first step to be taken in establishing a security control system is to conduct a security audit to determine the hospital's individual security needs. This audit should be conducted in consultation with a recognized outside security consultant or security director from another hospital who can objectively look at the hospital's security needs.

As soon as the hospital's security needs are identified, a set of written operational policies should be established. These written policies must be equally adhered to by all hospital employees. It becomes imperative, therefore, to publicize these policies so that all concerned individuals are aware of the hospital's rules and regulations. It should also be noted at this time that all employees, regardless of position, will be treated as equals and that all violations will be enforced to the full extent of the law.

Some proven effective preventive measures or controls within hospitals follow.

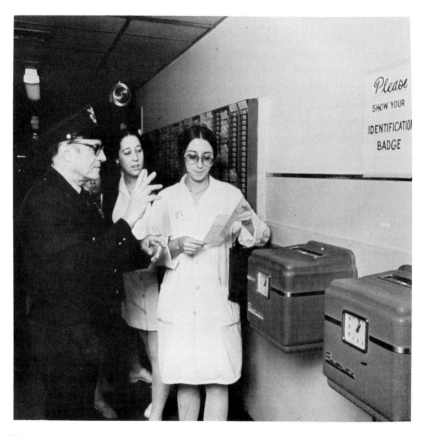

Figure 6. Employees should be required to enter and exit the hospital at a designated centralized location that is manned by a security officer. Each employee is responsible for punching out his or her own time card. (*Courtesy of* Frontier Security, Inc.)

1. Employees should be required to enter and exit the hospital at a designated location manned by a security officer.
2. A centralized time clock should be located at the designated employee entrance/exit.
3. All packages should be subject to inspection.

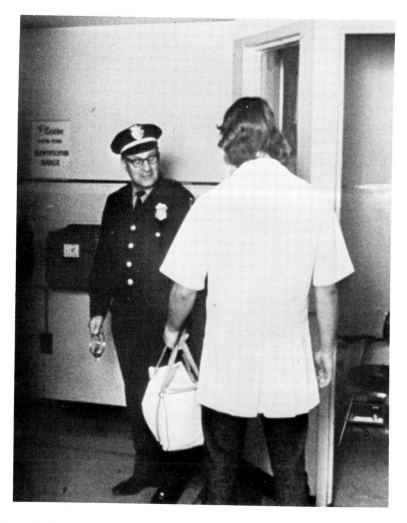

Figure 7. All packages should be subject to inspection. (*Courtesy of* Frontier Security, Inc.)

4. A package-pass system should be utilized to control material being removed from hospital premises.

5. All employees should park in the designated employee parking areas.

6. The use of visitor and vendor passes will enable the hospital to maintain a systematic control of the number of authorized people within the hospital complex.

7. The adoption of a policy that requires patients' valuables to be sent home with relatives and friends will help to reduce the loss of patients' valuables.

8. A procedure, such as a "valuables envelope" deposited with the business office, should be developed to protect the patients' valuables retained in the hospital.

9. A key control system should be adopted that restricts the number of master and submaster keys to a definite "need basis" only.

10. A room should be set aside within the security department to centralize all key making, locking equipment, and key control storage.

11. All hospital employees (doctors, nurses, technicians, volunteers, etc.) should be required to wear specially prepared name badges whenever they are at the hospital on official business.

12. Anti-intrusion alarm systems can be set up to protect merchandise stored in remote areas of the hospital complex.

13. Frequent security surveillance via a roving patrol that does not adhere to a rigid pattern for their rounds can be utilized.

14. Maintain accurate inventory control. Utilize certified public accountants — not internal accountants — to supervise annual inventories.

15. Develop a system for periodic unannounced physical inventories.

16. Develop a system of controls at the receiving dock that includes a detailed accounting for all incoming materials at the dock and a detailed verification by another source at the storage area.

17. Restrict pedestrian traffic at the dock so as not to encourage pilferage of temporary unattended materials.
18. The use of a well-planned, integrated security system that utilizes closed-circuit television and other supporting electronic equipment enables the hospital security force to provide maximum surveillance of trouble spots, such as the pharmacy area where narcotics are stored, out of the way storage areas, and the heavy traffic area of the gift shop.
19. Utilize effective lighting of exterior and interior areas as a preventive measure to deter theft and protect hospital personnel and property.
20. Foremost in importance to effective security control is the need to have a *well-trained* security force that is backed up by management.

The controls listed are not all-inclusive. They are meant to be an overview of hospital security. Many of these controls are further expanded in individual units of this text for greater depth and clarity. Experience and additional training will hopefully fill in any missing gaps.

SELECTED READINGS

Bishop, Vernon R.: Choose the right protective lighting arrangement. *Plant Engineering*, October 1964.

Burstein, Harvey: Reducing the Problem of Pilferage. *Hospitals, 31*:54-55, September 16, 1957.

Cole, A. G.: Employee Dishonesty. *Hospital Accounting, 22*:25-26, February 1968.

Colling, Russell: How One Hospital Developed Its Top-rated Security Program. *Hospitals Topics,* 29-33, July 1969.

Colling, Russell: *Hospital Security.* Los Angeles, Security World Publishing Co. Inc., 1976.

Glassman, Stanley A. and Fitzgerald, William J.: Contemporary Changes That Improve Your Hospital's Security. *Security World, II*, 9:30-35, October 1974.

Heller, Harry: Loss Prevention is Aim of Security Program. *Modern Hospital, 103*, No. 1:85, July 1964.

Hemphill, Charles F., Jr.: Limiting Loss Potential From Employee Theft. *Security World, 12*(2):28-29, February 1975.

Hospital Security. *Today's Hospital,* 2:2-4, 19, July 1965.

Internal Theft. Los Angeles, Security World Publishing Co. Inc.

Jaspan, Norman: Preventive Management — Cure For Hospital Dishonesty. *Hospital Topics.*

Jaspan, Norman: Why Employees Steal. *U. S. News and World Report,* 70:78-82, May 3, 1971.

Jaspan, Norman: *Mind Your Own Business.* Englewood Cliffs, P-H, 1974.

Jaspan, Norman: *Thieves On The Payroll.* New York, Investigations, Inc., Division of Norman Jaspan Associates, Inc., 1968.

Jorgensen, R. E.: Securing The Movement of Material. *Security Management,* November 1975.

Kingsbury, Arthur A.: *Introduction to Security and Crime Prevention Surveys.* Springfield, Thomas, 1973.

McLean, James C.: Is Your Hospital Being Robbed? *Modern Hospital, 103,* No. 1:79-82 and 150, July 1964.

Mitchell, Ian H.: An Internal Review Can Help In Recognizing Security Needs. *Hospital Administration — Canada,* October 1968.

Nelson, Benjamin O.: Effective Controllers Guard Dollar Security. *Modern Hospital, 103,* No. 1:95-96, July 1964.

Palmer, Robert: How North Memorial Hospital Solves These 12 Major Security Problems. *Modern Hospital,* 65-67, December 1971.

Post, Richard C.: *Determining Security Needs.* Madison, Oak Security Publication Division, 1973.

Rosenbaum, Richard W.: Can We Predict Employee Theft? *Security World,* 12(9):26-104, October 1975.

Security Guidelines For Hospitals, The Greater New York Hospital Association, New York, 1968.

Toepfer, Edwin F.: Are Your Doors "Wide Open" To Burglary? *Buildings,* 57:48-50, August 1963.

Chapter 7

PATROLS

The Importance of Good Patrolling

THE "backbone" of any good security opera-
tion is the officers' awareness and adherence to good patrol
procedures. It is through a thorough understanding of patrol
functions that criminal actions are deterred and safety hazards
are corrected. Webster's Seventh New Collegiate Dictionary de-
fines patrol as "the action of traversing a district or beat . . . for
the purpose of observing or of the maintenance of security."

A key word in Webster's definition is "observing." A security
officer must be constantly alert to details as he patrols his post.
He should always be able to spot things that are out of place or
unusual. His power of observation can help prevent a tragedy
and/or a criminal activity. Observation is a result of intelligent
curiosity that includes the utilization of all the senses, which
can and should be developed by all security officers.

THINGS TO WATCH FOR WHILE ON PATROL

While patrolling an area, guards should be careful to observe
the following:

(1) Doors and windows in buildings that are not secure
should be secured with any means at hand, and notification
through the proper channels should follow. A search of the
premises should always be conducted in an area that has been
found improperly secured.

(2) Suspicious persons or known criminals found loitering
should be carefully observed. Persons with no apparent destina-
tion or purpose, as well as unauthorized persons, should be
directed to leave the premises.

(3) Guards should watch closely for signs of disorder, excite-
ment, or unusual activity, such as large groups of people,
drunk or quarrelsome persons, or persons running away or

towards some incident or location.

(4) Conditions which are hazardous or require actions such as the repair of sidewalks, fire hazards, or safety hazards should be reported without delay. In some instances, guards may be required to take some remedial action until a more permanent repair can be accomplished. Safety hazards to be sought out and reported include:

1. Broken windows not only provide drafts and possible cuts but also provide easy access to the premises to unauthorized personnel.
2. Leaky or open water faucets not only cost the hospital needless money but can also present a safety hazard — slippery floors.
3. Defective electrical wiring or overloaded circuits not only cause short circuits but, more importantly might lead to a potential fire and loss of life.
4. Uncapped and unattended inflammables, such as oil cans, gas cans, and open paints, should not only be capped but should be removed to a safe storage place.
5. No smoking regulations, especially in areas that have oxygen in use, should be strictly enforced. Oxygen supports combustion — it does not burn by itself.
6. Cracked walking surfaces, such as sidewalks and steps, should be immediately reported in order that they may be fixed. Remember that broken sidewalks and steps lead to trips, slips, and falls.

The lists of physical hazards are too numerous to mention in any great detail. It is strongly suggested that the security office work hand-in-hand with the hospital safety committee (see Chapter 21). Always remember, the security officer is often the eyes and ears of the hospital administrative staff. Guards should immediately report anything noticed that may cause an injury.

MAKING ROUNDS WITH A RECORDING
OR WATCH-TOUR CLOCK

Many fire insurance carriers require that at least four tours of

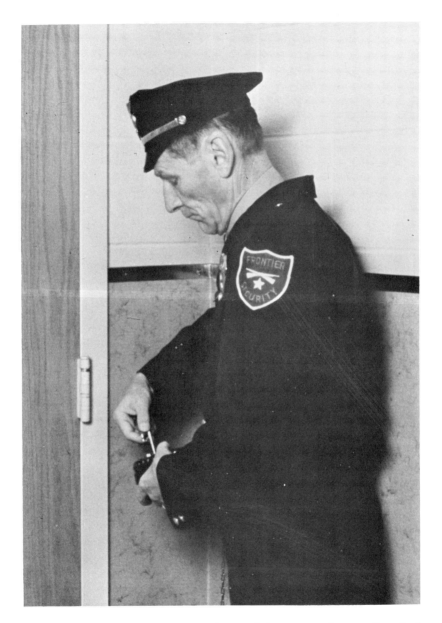

Figure 8. A security officer records his rounds by means of a recording clock. (*Courtesy of* Frontier Security, Inc.)

the hospital be made every twenty-four hour period. In order to provide proof that the rounds were made, some security officers are assigned a fixed patrol route that requires them to record their movements by means of a recording clock. A recording clock uses a sequence of strategically located keys throughout the hospital that enables paper discs, locked inside the clock, to be punched or imprinted with the corresponding number of the key when it is inserted and turned.

The keys are housed in small metal containers that are securely mounted in numerous locations throughout the hospital that map out the route the security officer must take in completing his rounds. The officer assigned this route should have at his disposal a set of instructions that spell out the path to be taken and the exact location of each key. (See the sample of a possible "Recording Key Locations Map" in the chapter Appendix.)

The security officer's tour of duty (see sample in the chapter Appendix) will indicate the designated hours for conducting the clock tours. Most insurance carriers prefer them to be made during the late evening hours. In any case, the clock rounds

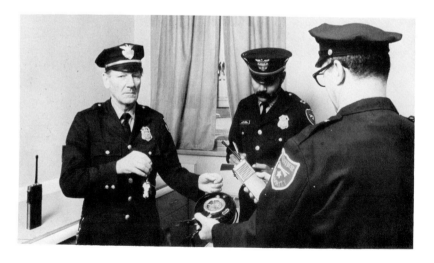

Figure 9. Keys, watch clock, and radio transceiver are transferred as the patrol tour changes. (*Courtesy of* Frontier Security, Inc.)

provide a recorded tape that proves that rounds were made during a particular period of time.

PATROLLING THE PERIMETER (OUTSIDE) OF THE HOSPITAL

The main function of the "outside" perimeter patrol should be to provide adequate security of the hospital complex and to protect persons entering or exiting the hospital facilities. The security officer, therefore, will be responsible for all locking and unlocking procedures that normally occur during his tour of duty. He will be responsible for physically checking to see that all exterior doors and chains that should be locked are locked at the proper times.

The outside perimeter patrol will include:

1. Checking isolated areas for unlawful entry or other irregularities.
2. Controlling and regulating pedestrian and vehicular traffic at the hospital complex.
3. Checking areas surrounding the nursing quarters, especially during the evening hours, for persons loitering there.
4. Checking ground floor windows and entrances.
5. Checking the receiving areas.
6. Insuring that fire lanes are kept free of parked automobiles.
7. Insuring that emergency room ambulance parking areas are clear of unauthorized vehicles.
8. Checking staff parking areas for proper vehicle passes or decals.
9. Patrolling visitor and staff parking lots to deter car thefts and muggings.
10. Providing night escort service.
11. Checking to see that all outdoor protective lighting along the hospital's perimeter and between the hospital's passage ways are operable.
12. Patrolling the entire hospital including the detached buildings such as the power plant, laundry, nursing

quarters, etc.

Night Escort Service

Mugging and rape incident rates are especially high during the evening hours. Employees entering and exiting a hospital complex during late evening hours can be a prime target for the criminal. For this reason, the hospital security force should

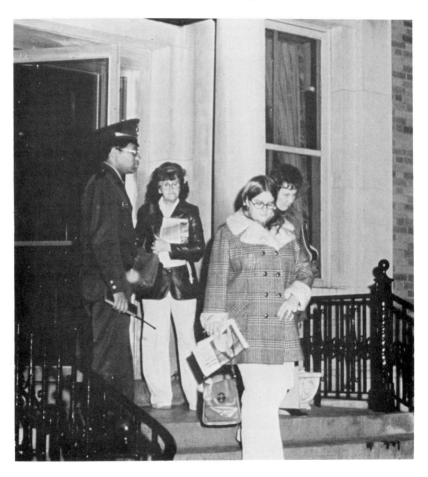

Figure 10. Security officer escorts nurses from the nursing quarters to the hospital. (*Courtesy of* Frontier Security, Inc.)

provide an evening escort service that patrols, either by foot or by vehicles, the areas to and from the nursing quarters, the hospital and the parking lots, and designated areas, as requested.

When a security patrol vehicle is assigned to the escort service, it does not necessarily mean that security officers will drive the hospital personnel to and from buildings or to their cars. This is optional to individual hospitals. Whatever the policy of the hospital, the night escort service should provide protection for all employees while they are in the process of going to and from the hospital complex.

TWENTY-FOUR HOUR ROVING PATROLS

Several security officers, in uniform and/or in plainclothes, should be assigned to patrol the hospital complex on unscheduled rounds. While patrolling, these security officers should be "systematically unsystematic."

The "roving security officer should not do the same thing at

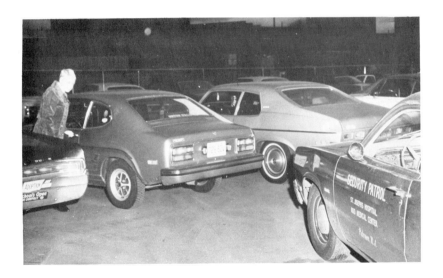

Figure 11. The security patrol provides staff protection while going to and from the hospital complex. (*Courtesy of* Frontier Security, Inc.)

the same time every day. He should constantly change his routine. He should maneuver so as to observe people and locations without, in turn, being observed. He should keep an eye on employees, patients, and visitors. Anything suspicious should be reported, no matter how slight. Through constant vigilance and unpredicted appearances, he can generate a psychological effect that would deter potential offenders from committing acts of vandalism and theft.

Other duties assigned to this position would be to answer all security assistance calls, to perform the duties of an investigator as the need arises, and to assume a supervisory role of the security officers assigned to his tour.

APPENDIX

Recording Clock Key Locations
(Sample)

KEY	*LOCATION*	*INSTRUCTIONS*
1	Laboratory Hallway	Laboratory Hallway is located next to the X-ray Dept. midway between the main lobby and the emergency entrance. The key is located across from the Chemistry and Microbiology rooms.
2	Record Room	Walk down hall — turn left through double doors past X-ray Dept. — across hallway by turning right and left to stairwell which is by the main bank of elevators — downstairs and left at bottom. Walk straight to end of hall — turn right and go to end of hallway. Open door to Record Room. Key is located straight ahead on right hand side next to office door.
3	Receiving Room	Walk back out of Record Room — straight down hall until you reach double doors to Receiving Room (located on left side of hall). Open door and turn right. Walk past second door on right — next to filing cabinet is key on the right side of wall.
4	Kitchen	Walk back out double doors — go straight to kitchen entrance (on left side of hall) (double doors) open door and walk straight back to end of kitchen — below exit sign is key box.
5	Clinic (Left Side)	Walk back out kitchen, turn left and walk past Pharmacy (check this area) at end of hallway turn left. Go to last door on right. Open door to Physical Therapy Dept. Turn left to Tank Room — go through big door on left and then go right. Key is just inside first door on right. (Check all rooms in Physical Therapy).
6	Linen Room	Walk back out of Physical Therapy — turn left at end of hall — walk up ramp, open door — continue straight — linen room is located on left side of corridor — open door and walk into second room. Key box is on fourth brick pillar.
7	Maintenance Room	Return to hall — turn left and walk about 50 ft. down on left side of corridor is the Maintenance entrance. Open door and proceed etc.

Tour V Duty Assignment
(12 M to 8:30 AM)

12 M to 1:30 AM	Patrol emergency entrance
1:30 AM to 2:30 AM	Make internal check of entire building including all nursing floors
2:30 AM to 3:00 AM	Patrol emergency entrance
3:00 AM to 4:00 AM	Clock tour
4:00 AM to 4:30 AM	Meal break
4:30 AM to 5:30 AM	Clock tour
5:30 AM to 6:30 AM	Patrol emergency area
6:30 AM to 7:30 AM	Raises flag. Unlock doors to Clinic, old emergency ramp, Maintenance-Receiving, main lobby, linen room (sliding doors). Take cones from reserved spaces and place them around building in main lobby area and administration bldg.
7:30 AM to 8:30 AM	Patrol between emergency entrance and main lobby. Complete daily reports.

Supervising Guards Daily Assignment Record

DATE:_____   SHIFT: _____

REPORT OF:_____   GUARDS ON DUTY: _____

DUTY ASSIGNMENT	FROM	TO	REMARKS	FROM	TO	REMARKS
Briefing and Inspection of Men and Equipment						
Internal check of buildings						
External check — Buildings and Grounds						
Visitor Control — Main Lobby						
Traffic Control						
Parking Control						
Watch Clock Tours						
Emergency Area						
Investigations*						
Special Assignments						
Administrative Reports & Duties						

Signature: _____

Comments: _____

_____

_____

_____

_____

*INVESTIGATIONS OF ACCIDENTS OR INCIDENTS REQUIRE SPECIAL RE-
PORTS.

SELECTED READINGS

Colling, Russell E.: It's the Hard Day's Night of the Security Force that Creates Safe Setting For Patient Care. *Modern Hospital, 110*(1):69-70, January 1968.

Collins, William P.: Physical Security Planning. *Police Chief:* 247-251, October 1970.

Howington, Jon: Prevention and enforcement concepts of the patrol function for security officers. *Security Education Briefs* (OAK Security Inc.), *2*(No. 1):

The Police Administration and Public Safety College of Social Science, Michigan State University: *Law and Order Training for Civil Defense Emergency, Student Manual* (Part B). East Lansing, Mich St U Pr, August 1965.

Mitchell, Eleanor: Night Safety — A Problem for Nurses. *The Canadian Nurse, 66*:28-30, February 1970.

—— Patrol Concepts for security officers. *Security Education Briefs* (OAK Security Inc.), *2*(No. 2):

—— Patrol techniques for security officers. *Security Education Briefs* (OAK Security Inc.), *2*(No. 8):

Security Guidelines For Hospitals, The Greater New York Hospital Association, New York, 1968.

Whipperman, Robert F.: The ABC's of private patrol. *Security World, 2*(No. 4): June 1965.

Chapter 8

KEY CONTROL SYSTEM

THE problem of providing easy access within a hospital complex, while at the same time providing a security system for controlling keys, is one that plagues most hospital security departments. In this unit, the authors will outline some basic steps to a workable key control system. The system that will be initiated at your hospital will depend upon your specific needs.

The important aspect to be considered in this unit is the development of a standard key policy whose control rests with the hospital security department. Essential to a key control system is a safe and sturdy key cabinet. An index should be maintained for all issued keys and this index should be further backed-up by custody receipts. If feasible, a room should be set aside within the security department to centralize all key making, locking equipment, and key control storage.

Keys should be issued to authorized personnel on an individual lock basis whenever possible, even if it becomes necessary to issue several keys for different locks. A cross reference file should be maintained on all keys and personnel holding keys. The system should include the keys to desks, file cabinets, lockers, etc. Hospital personnel should have to sign a form that states they will not loan their issued keys to anyone and that they will immediately report any loss or theft of keys to the security department. The hospital should adopt a policy that requires employees to turn in keys to the security department when employees are transferred or leave. Keys should also be turned in to the security department when employees are on vacation. Locks should be changed when security is breached.

Periodically, the security department should conduct an "audit" whereby authorized personnel must produce keys to ensure that the keys have not been lost or stolen. A further control is to have a specific design imprinted on the bow of the key that will identify the key as being an official, original issue hospital key.

The key should also have engraved on it "Do Not Duplicate." The Hospital's name need not be imprinted on the key since the key will already have a logo, a specific design, that will identify the key as being that of the hospital.

The issuance of submaster keys should be based on a definite "need basis" and only to those individuals who have to operate a large number of locks in a particular area. The issuance of grand master keys should be kept to an absolute minimum. Grand master keys should be restricted to top management people who have a definite need for such a key. These individuals should be required to sign a receipt for its issuance. Needless to say, these individuals should be cautioned about lending these keys to anyone. Once a master key has been duplicated by an unauthorized person, it becomes impossible to know the degree of security remaining in the lock system. The cost of regaining good security after the system has been compromised could be very costly, not only in terms of dollars but also in terms of waste of materials and labor involved.

The practice of leaving a master key at the switchboard, admittance office, or information desk for the convenience of people who get locked out or who forget their keys is a dangerous one. Simply signing for the key is not the answer. A good practice for master key control is to restrict it to the security officer on duty. He will be charged with the responsibility of admitting authorized personnel to a specific area. Even then, the person desiring entry to a locked area should produce proper hospital identification (see the unit on employee identification) and a valid reason for wishing to enter the area. The sign-in procedure, noting the exact time of entry and exit, should be recorded in the security officer's daily log. This procedure is especially applicable after normal working hours. (See Appendix this chapter for sample form.)

CARD ACCESS SYSTEMS

A card key is a plastic magnetically coded card that resembles, in size and shape, a standardized credit card. It can be magnetically coded to operate any number or combination of access controls — even if each has a different code combination. Locks are programmed by means of a specially coded plastic matrix card. Codes may be changed without removal of locks by simply inserting a new matrix card. Any issued card, therefore, may be invalidated instantly in case of loss or theft.

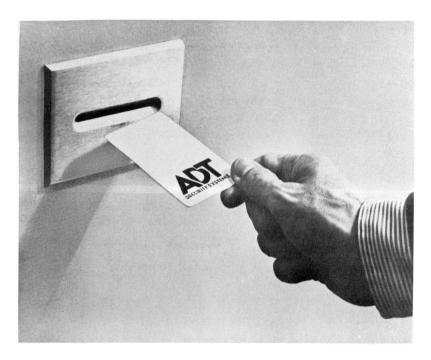

Figure 12. A card access system for limiting entry to pharmacy areas, storerooms, and other critical locations within the hospital. (*Courtesy of* ADT Security Systems.)

The card key system can be dual coded to permit personnel access only during assigned shifts. It additionally permits customized printing and the permanent attachment of a photograph to the card for employee identification.

The magnetically encoded card can be interfaced with a pushbutton array. Entry would then be obtained by insertion of the proper access card into the pushbutton unit's slot and pushing a series of buttons in a predetermined sequence. Pushbutton codes can be changed by authorized personnel in sixty seconds. The system can also interface with a silent alarm to indicate an improper entry attempt.

The card key system is very versatile. The system permits mastering (pass-key) and submastering (limited access), a feature to prevent card "pass back" from one person to another, a voiding and data print out feature, and controlled access to a parking area.

LOCKS AND COMBINATIONS

Door locks should be of a good quality tumbler type, preferably of the tamper proof variety. A lock that has a removable core is strongly recommended. The combination on these locks can be easily reset whenever a key is lost or stolen. A special key is used with these locks that removes the core so that they can be interchanged with another.

Hospitals are usually equipped with a large number of employee lockers. The combination type locks are preferable for lockers because the combinations may easily be changed to coincide with personnel changes. It is much simpler, less costly, and safer to issue a new combination rather than a key to new employees.

A good key control system is the by-product of good planning and the headaches that accompany a complex key system can be minimized if the security of the system remains intact.

APPENDIX

Record of Keys Issued

RECORD OF KEYS ISSUED											MONTH		
	I.D. NUMBER	KEY NUMBER	ISSUED			RETURNED		
NAME			DATE	TIME	GUARD	DATE	TIME	GUARD

SELECTED READINGS

Bilhorn, Robert: Card key access control at Chicago convention. *Industrial Security*, December 1968.

Crichton, W.: *Practical Course In Modern Locksmithing*. Chicago, Nelson-Hall, 1957.

Eskin, David H.: Lock and key control and master keying. *Industrial Security*, December 1964.

Grumback, A. T.: Locks and Locking — Security Destruction By Masterkey. *Security World, 12*(9):40, October 1975.

Haswell, William S.: Lock and key control and master keying — a neglected area of security. *Industrial Security*, December 1964.

Johnstone, Theodore H.: Lock and key control and master keying. *Industrial Security*, December 1964.

Lynk, Leo: Establishing an easy access security system. *Building Maintenance and Modernization*, May 1969. (Appears in *Hospital Security and Safety Journal Articles*. Flushing, Med Exam, 1969.)

Robinson, Robert L.: Decision to masterkey, Part I. *Security World*, July/August 1974.

———: Masterkeying — the decision to masterkey, Part II, *Security World* II, #9: October 1974.

Tobia, Marc Weber: *Locks, Safes, and Security*. Springfield, Thomas, 1971.

Toepfer, Edwin F.: A new-building look at locks and keys. *Security World*, II, No. 10:20-22, November 1974.

———: The door that locks must go on. *Security World*, II (No. 10):50-54, November, 1974.

———: Lock security: cylinders, keys and keying, part I. *Security World, 2* (No. 5): July-August, 1965.

———: Lock security: cylinders, keys and keying, part II. *Security World, 2* (No. 6): September, 1965.

Trends in lock and key design. *Security Gazette*, October 1961.

Walsh, Timothy J.: A machine record method for maintaining lock and key accountability. *Industrial Security*, April 1965.

Underwriters Laboratories, Inc.: *Combination Locks*. Chicago, National Board of Fire Underwriters, 1961.

Chapter 9

PERSONNEL CONTROL

IDENTIFICATION

IT has been stated numerous times throughout this text that the security officer's primary concern within the hospital complex is the protection of life and property. The responsibility to keep unauthorized persons from the hospital complex is also an important concern. A hospital is in operation twenty-four hours a day, with employees coming and going throughout the day. Without a system of employee identification, virtually anyone can come and go as they please. When that happens, security becomes an impossible task. A simple, not too expensive system of identification is to require all hospital employees, including doctors, nurses, technicians, volunteers, management, security, and clerical workers to wear specially prepared name badges whenever they are at the hospital on official business. The name badges could be color coded to distinguish between employee classifications. The name badges should be distinctive enough so unauthorized people can not easily purchase them in an ordinary stationary shop. The hospital's name and/or logo should be included on the badge along with the name and title of the individual. An employee photo can be included on the badge. The name badge should be a clip-on badge required to be worn at all times while on the premises. The policy on wearing name badges serves a dual purpose in that it identifies authorized hospital personnel and identifies by exception all others, e.g. patients, visitors, vendors. The real significance of wearing a name badge is that it enables the hospital staff to readily distinguish people who are authorized personnel from those people who may not be there on legitimate hospital business. From a security standpoint, this is invaluable. In addition to the hospital security staff, all supervisory personnel should be authorized to politely ask anyone in the hospital for proper identification.

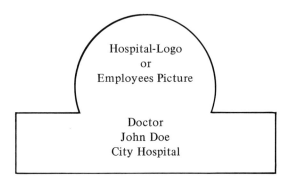

Figure 13. Sample of a name badge to be worn by all hospital employees.

Identification Card

A backup procedure to the name badge is the employee identification card. All hospital employees should be issued a lami-
nated identification card. If a photo is used on both the
identification card and the name badge, they both should be
printed, if possible, from the same negative. This will provide
security with an easy visual comparison. The identification
card should contain the following information:

(a) Name
(b) Height and weight
(c) I. D. # or Social Security #
(d) Color of eyes and hair
(e) Fingerprint
(f) Photo
(g) Employee's signature

A procedure should be developed to provide a temporary name
badge for employees who leave their badges at home or for any
other reason arrive at the hospital without their name badge.
Security should have a central employee file index at their
disposal to check employee signatures and/or photos. Once
positive identification has been made for an employee who has
forgotten his name badge, a temporary badge can be issued.

Employees should immediately report a lost or stolen name
badge or identification card to security. When an employee

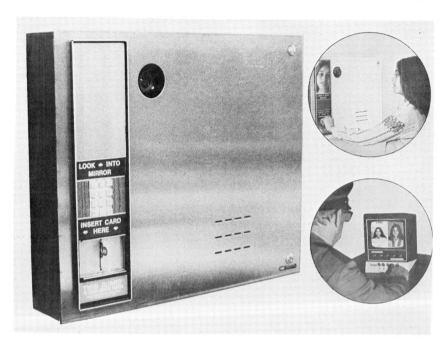

Figure 14. The security officer sees a sharp picture of the person desiring entrance and a close-up image of their identification card. The security officer allows or denies access. (*Courtesy of* Visual Methods Incorporated.)

terminates his employment, the identification card and the name badge should be returned to the security department.

If the security department wishes to retain all employee name badges at a central location within the hospital, a pass-badge system can be used. Employees entering a central fixed post would present their identification card to the security officer who would issue the employee's badge. All badges should be filed in either alphabetical or numerical order by job function to help alleviate bottlenecks (as security searches for the proper employee badge). Upon exiting the hospital, from the same central fixed post, employees would return their name badges to the security officer on duty. The pass-badge system provides a tight security control of hospital employees, since they are forced to identify themselves to the security officer upon entering and exiting the hospital.

The type of identification system that is ultimately employed

ST. JOSEPH'S HOSPITAL
AND MEDICAL CENTER, PATERSON, N.J.

_____
NAME

EMPLOYEE NO.

_____
DEPARTMENT

_____
SOCIAL SECURITY NO.

_____
EMPLOYEE SIGNATURE

ADMINISTRATOR

THIS IS YOUR OFFICIAL IDENTIFICATION

When embossed it entitles you to
FREE PARKING

It is non-transferable and must be carried
with you at all times. You must show your
I.D. when requested while on hospital
property.

You must return card to Security Dept.
on termination.

INSERT THIS END
THIS SIDE UP

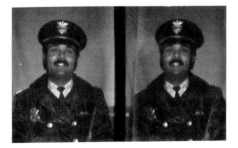

Figure 15. A sample of an identification card.

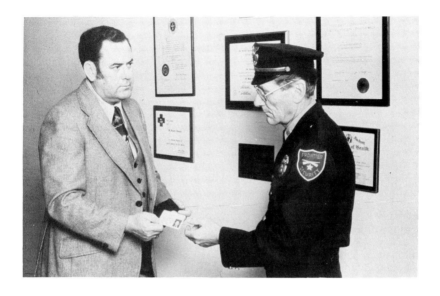

Figure 16. Security officer checks employee identification card for positive identification. (*Courtesy of* Frontier Security, Inc.)

will depend upon the hospital's size and security needs. All hospital employees must be thoroughly familiar with the system used. Further, security officers must enforce the identification regulations diligently and courteously.

SELECTED READINGS

Exit control system helps hospital cut pilferage, vandalism. *American Hospital Products*, 4, 17, March 1968.

Norpell, Bradley F.: Identification cards and badges. *Security World, 3 (No. 2): February 1966.*

Powell, Gregg E.: Identification cards: How to use them. *Security World, 12* (No. 2): 22-23, February 1975.

Strobl, W. M.: Hospital security: A security consultant's viewpoint. *Federal of American Hospitals Review, 3,* 38, Fall 1969.

Sullivan, Thomas J.: How the hospital can make internal control work. *Financial Management,* 3-6, October 1969.

Weber, Rudy: Selling security to employees. *Security World, 4* (No. 4): April 1967.

Chapter 10

PACKAGE PASS SYSTEM

E VERY hospital should have a system to control packages and materials being removed from hospital premises. A system that has met with success in many hospitals is a "Package Pass" system. All employees desiring to remove packages or parcels from the hospital premises are required to surrender a package pass to the security officer at a fixed security check point upon leaving.

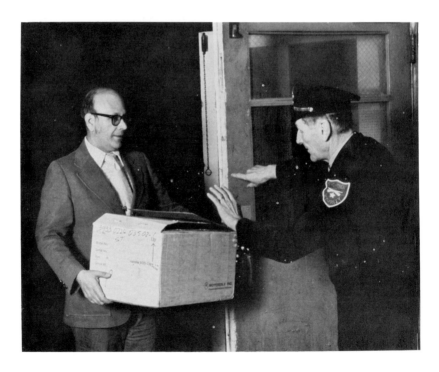

Figure 17. Security officers are instructed not to allow any hospital property to be removed from the hospital without written approval of the appropriate authorizing administrator. (*Courtesy of* Frontier Security, Inc.)

All hospital employees should be required to enter and exit the hospital through a specific fixed security check point. This fixed security check post should be used by employees reporting for duty, while on duty, exiting their shift, or merely visiting. Requiring one entrance-exit designation will enable the security officer to maintain control on the package pass system.

Passes should not be required for personal property which can be easily identified, such as shoes, sweaters, purses, or umbrellas. Passes should be required for items identified as hospital property; written approval of the appropriate authorizing administrator is necessary. Any item not covered by a package pass and identified as hospital property should be confiscated by the security officer.

The security officers will submit to the security department all passes which have been collected. All passes will be checked with issuing departments daily to insure accuracy. A signature card should be readily available to security officers for comparison.

If hospital property is loaned to an employee or to another hospital the package pass procedure is as follows:

1. The department director issues a package pass to the employee.
2. The original copy is given to the employee with the package and surrendered to the security officer upon exit.
3. The second copy is sent by the department director to the director of security, which is maintained on file.
4. The third copy is retained by the department director. Upon return of the loaned property, the department director notes such return on his copy of the package pass and forwards it to the security department.

APPENDIX

Package Pass

NO._____

Date Issued_____

POLICY:

This Package Pass must be used by all persons whenever any property is to be taken from the hospital premises. It must be surrendered to the security officer stationed at the main lobby entrance upon leaving the hospital.

NOTE: A package pass is not required for personal belongings or attire such as shoes, sweaters, umbrellas, purses, uniforms, etc. However, the security officer is authorized to examine *any* package.

NAME:_____DEPARTMENT:_____

Description and number of items including identification or serial number, if applicable:

_____

_____

_____

_____

_____   _____

Immediate Supervisor's Signature   Date

If a package contains hospital property (e.g. typewriters, visual aid equipment, medical equipment, etc.) the package pass must be approved by the appropriate assistant administrator.

_____   _____

Assistant Administrator's Signature   Date

FOR SECURITY OFFICER'S USE:

Departure Date: _____   Time: _____

_____
Security Officer's Signature

_____

Loaned hospital property returned on _____ at _____
                                        Date   Time

_____
Immediate Supervisor's Signature

                    RETAIN COPIES AS FOLLOWS:

                    PINK COPY - Employee
                    GREEN COPY - Security Dept.
                    WHITE COPY - Immediate Supvr.

Courtesy of St. Joseph's Hospital and Medical Center, Paterson, New Jersey.

SELECTED READINGS

Cary, Fred W.: Property pass systems — a deterrent to internal theft. *Security Management, 19*(5):18-22, November 1975.

Leydon, Joseph L.: Salesman's pass aids security and product selection. *Modern Hospital,* August 1968.

Telfer, George A.: Internal control for inventory and property. *Financial Management,* 27-30, October 1969.

Chapter 11

EMPLOYEE PARKING CONTROL

ALL hospital employees should be advised that parking on the hospital complex is at the owner's risk. The hospital does not normally assume liability for employee vehicles that are damaged or stolen while parked on the hospital premises. Employees should, therefore, be cautioned when leaving their parked vehicle to close all windows, leave no objects of value visible in the car, lock all car doors, and take their keys with them.

Employee Vehicle Registration

All vehicles parked on hospital property by employees must be registered with the hospital security department. The employee registration information should include:

Employee's full name and mailing address.
Position at the hospital.
Hospital department telephone number.
Description of employee's vehicle as to make, model, color, year.
The vehicle's license plate number.
The owner's driver's license number.
Description and information on employee's second vehicle if used for work.

The employee vehicle registration form should be cross-filed by name and license plate number. Upon completion of the registration form, a decal that authorizes the employee to park in a designated parking area should be issued.

Parking Regulations

A parking decal should be issued to all hospital staff who have registered their vehicle with the security department. Employee parking would be restricted to the designated area indicated on the parking decal. Employee parking decals, therefore, should be coded by color, numbers, or letters to coincide with the specific designated parking area.

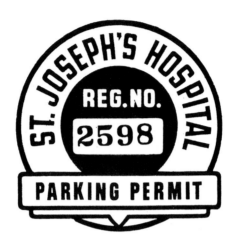

Figure 18.

The parking decal should be displayed on a designated location of the vehicle, e.g. the upper left hand corner of the window on the driver's side. If an employee often drives another vehicle to work, additional decals should be available. Employees should be required to scrape off their decals when selling or exchanging their vehicles. The scrapings should be returned to the security department and a new decal issued upon updating the employee's vehicle registration form.

A procedure should be established whereby the personnel department notifies the security department of an employee's termination. The employee's vehicle registration file should be pulled and the employee should return the scraped decal to the security department as part of the hospital separation procedure.

Additional instructions to employees regarding parking privileges should include the following:

- •All parking is under the direction and control of the security department. Please obey signs and the instructions of the security officers. It is their responsibility to keep order.
- •Vehicles must be parked according to plan.
- •Perpendicular parking only is permitted.
- •Please remember that in the interest of hospital safety, access to fire lanes must be kept open at all times. Vehicles that are illegally parked create safety hazards and, if necessary, will be removed from the property at the owner's expense.
- •Employees other than those assigned are NOT permitted to park in the following reserved areas:

(a) Doctor's Parking Lot
(b) Patient Discharge area
(c) Emergency Room Receiving areas

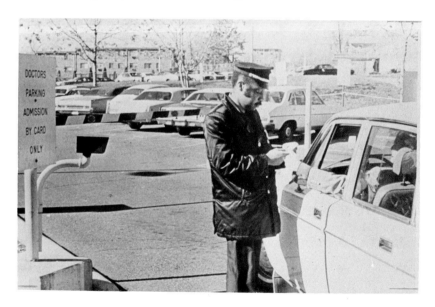

Figure 19. Security officer checks identification card for admittance into the "Restricted to Doctors Only" parking area. (*Courtesy of* Frontier Security, Inc.)

(d) Delivery and Receiving areas
(e) Any other area designated to be a reserved area and posted accordingly

"Security's Report of Parking Violations" in the chapter Appendix should be used to report employee-owned cars only. Visitors must be handled by paging and/or police action when necessary. If a car is not registered with the hospital but is known to be employee owned, establish the identity of the owner, issue a decal, and report any subsequent violations.

Parking and traffic regulation signs should be posted in all appropriate locations to inform employees and visitors of the hospital parking regulations. When someone violates the parking regulations, they should be officially notified. A "Parking Notice" form (see chapter Appendix), can be used by security as a warning notice. If the situation warrants a traffic ticket and the security department is not empowered to issue one, the local police department should be notified.

Investigation of Cars Reported Stolen from Hospital Property

The format to follow in investigating reported stolen cars follows.

Accompany the complainant to the area from where the car was allegedly stolen. Make a physical check of the parking area for several reasons:

1. Make sure the car was actually stolen.
2. Determine if, in his haste, the thief dropped anything that might be used to identify him. (This sometimes happens.)
3. Question anyone sitting in a parked car in the vicinity. They may be able to furnish a physical description of the thief.

Complete an incident report obtaining all pertinent information. Establish approximate time, exact location, and whether or not the car was properly locked.

Advise the complainant to notify the police department as

soon as possible. If your investigation reveals any information or evidence that you think might be useful, report it to the police department and let them determine its value.

APPENDIX

Security's Report of Parking Violations

SECURITY'S REPORT OF PARKING VIOLATIONS

WEEK OF:_____ REPORT OF:_____

SECURITY OFFICERS INSTRUCTIONS: Beginning on Monday of each week, guards are required to keep a copy of this report with them in their daily rounds for the purpose of reporting employee owned vehicles illegally parked on Hospital property. A follow-up report to the appropriate Department Head will be sent from this office, so accuracy in reporting is most important. Reports should be submitted to the security office at the end of each normal week.

Date of Violation	Time	Location of Violation	Decal Number	License Number	Guard Action Was Car Moved?	Department Action-Report Sent?

Parking Notice

To provide the greatest convenience for the majority of people who use the hospital's parking area, it is necessary that ALL drivers follow the parking regulations and let courtesy and common sense be their guide.

Please cooperate with the security officer on duty, who is there to lend help and assistance.

Director Security

— — — — — — — — — — — — — —

IN THE FUTURE, PLEASE:

( ) Drive Slowly — 10 MPH or less — when on hospital property.
( ) Do not park in this area, it is reserved and so marked.
( ) Park carefully within the white lines to conserve parking spaces.
( ) Observe traffic signs. They are put there for a purpose.
( ) Do not park in roadway.
( ) Do not park here: This is an entrance, fire zone, loading zone.
( ) Park closer to the curb in order not to interfere with traffic.
( ) Perpendicular parking only.
( ) If you are an employee or someone authorized to park on hospital property, please REGISTER your vehicle at the security department as soon as possible. This will enable us to contact you immediately in case of an emergency. It also enables us to detect unauthorized use of our parking areas by outsiders.
( ) Other. . . . . . .

SELECTED READINGS

A Guide to Security Investigations. American Society For Industrial Security, Washington, D. C., 1970.

Downey, G. W.: Few rules for parking lot planning can help cut costs, irritation and nighttime danger. *Modern Nursing Home, 25*:43, August 1970.

Hospital parking. *Hospital Building Eng, 2*:29, May 1969.

Lomax, Joe B.: Parking lot security. *Security Education Briefs* (OAK Security Inc.), *2* (No. 4):

————:Parking security, Part II. *Security Education Briefs* (OAK Security Inc.), *2* (No. 5).:

Murphy, Harry J.: Security of Airport Parking Lots. *Security Management,* May 1975.

O'Flaherty, C. A.: Hospital parking. *Hospital Building Eng, 3*:9, May 1970.

Security Guidelines For Hospitals, The Greater New York Hospital Association, New York, 1968.

Chapter 12

GUIDELINES FOR SECURITY OFFICERS ASSIGNED TO THE EMERGENCY AREA

PERHAPS no other area of the hospital requires more control or attention than is required in the emergency service. A great deal of patience, understanding, and tact is necessary in order to properly deal with people who may not be functioning normally for a variety of reasons.

The emergency ward is a designated area of the hospital that is set up to handle critical situations that need immediate attention. Those who normally come to the emergency ward are either people in need of instantaneous medical aid or are the loved ones and friends of the patients being treated. The patients are there because of accidents, burns, cuts, drugs, alcohol, shock and other similar illnesses. They are usually accompanied by people who are interested in their safety and well being. In either case, the majority of people who come to the emergency ward are laboring under a physical or emotional strain.

The emergency ward is usually a busy area with traffic coming and going at all hours of the day. This area is usually more heavily traveled during the late evening hours when the normal visitor's entrances are closed and when the services rendered at private doctor's offices are unavailable. The emergency ward then becomes the primary entrance to the hospital for staff, patients, and visitors. In addition to handling emergency cases, the ward may also become the primary location for handling out-patient medical aid that cannot be secured from the closed private physician's office. The need for control of this area, therefore, is a top priority one.

In most hospitals, the emergency ward is a fixed post. The security officer who is usually assigned to this post must be

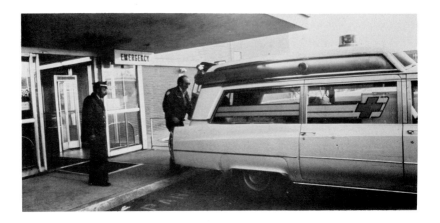

Figure 20. Security officer stands ready to lend assistance if needed to control vehicular and pedestrian traffic in the emergency area. (*Courtesy of* Frontier Security, Inc.)

sensitive to the anxieties and fears of the people who come to the emergency ward, while still maintaining control and order in line with his duties and responsibilities. He must know how to handle the intoxicated, the drug addict, the intruder, the press, and the family and friends of patients. Equally important, the security officer must always display courtesy, diplomacy, politeness, and respect.

Guidelines for Security Officers Assigned to Emergency Area

The primary function of the security officer on duty throughout the hospital shall be as follows:

1. Protection of life and property.
2. Preservation of the peace.
3. Prevention of vandalism and other crimes.
4. Prevention and detection of fire and other safety hazards.
5. Enforcement of hospital rules and regulations.

Specific Duties of the Security Officers Assigned to the Emergency Area

1. Render assistance with ambulance patients and anyone else requiring assistance to gain entrance to the hospital for the purpose of receiving emergency treatment.
2. Control vehicular and pedestrian traffic in the immediate area of the emergency entrance.
3. Restrict access to examination and treatment areas in accordance with existing hospital policies.
4. Complete "A Security Incident Report" on unusual events or incidents.
5. Perform other related duties as assigned by the director of security or as dictated by hospital policy.

It is vitally essential to establish a good working relationship between security personnel and the medical staff of the emergency service.

The proper role of the security officer on duty in the emergency area must be clearly defined and understood before we can hope to achieve the common goal of rendering the best possible assistance to patients.

Summary

Guidelines are established to promote efficient performance. They cannot possibly apply to all security problems, nor will they replace good judgment. They will, however, be of great assistance when used in conjunction with a "common sense" application of the rules.

SELECTED READINGS

Denny, Helen Finston: *Emergency Room And The Hospital Security Officer,* a paper presented at the Fifth Annual Institute For Hospital Security Guards, Greater New York Hospital Association, New York, 1971.
Young, Carl B.: First-Aid and Resuscitation. Springfield, Thomas, 1954.

Chapter 13

VISITOR CONTROL

O NE of the most difficult assignments facing
security in a hospital is good control of visitors. A *National
Survey on Hospital Security* by the Burns Security Institute in
1972 reported that the responding hospital administrators considered "visitor control the most formidable security problem

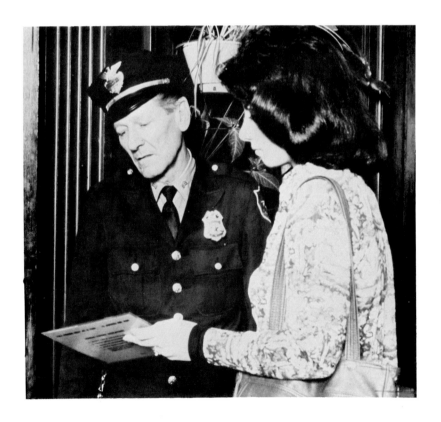

Figure 21. Security officer checks visitor pass. (*Courtesy of* Frontier Security,
Inc.)

that has to be overcome." The reasons complicating visitor control, the report continues, "are too many entrances and exits, multi-building complexes on huge acreage, unmanned entrance gates, absence of perimeter fencing and doors opened at unauthorized times."

All visitors to the hospital should be required to enter the hospital via the main entrance. They should then report to the security desk or a reception desk, where a visitor's pass will be issued to a specific patient's room. It is recommended that the number of visitors to a patient be limited to two at a time. This procedure will allow for a systematic control of the number of visitors per floor while providing the patient with a reasonable number of family and friends at a time.

Visitor Pass

Upon admittance of a patient to the hospital, a visitor's pass card should be prepared listing the patient's complete name, bed, and room number. This card should then be filed in alphabetical order and administered through the main security or reception desk. The cards should be color coded to coincide with specific floors and specific wards. The cards should also be of a large size, roughly five by seven inches, and difficult to fold to assist visitors in remembering to return the cards instead of casually placing them in their clothing or handbags.

The color code and relatively large size of the visitor's pass will enable the security officers and the hospital staff to easily recognize whether a visitor is or is not on the designated floor of the issued pass. If elevator operators are used in the hospital, the size and color of the pass will also assist them in directing the visitor to the proper location. Additional information to be incorporated on the visitor's pass includes:

(a) Name of the hospital.
(b) The specific location for which the pass is intended, e.g. pediatric ward, maternity ward, etc.
(c) Reminders — such as
    (1) No smoking in rooms with oxygen.
    (2) The visiting hour time schedule should be shown.

ST. JOSEPH'S HOSPITAL AND MEDICAL CENTER
703 Main Street
Paterson, New Jersey

VISITOR'S PASS

INTENSIVE CARE
PATIENTS

All Visitors Must Be At Least 14 Years Of Age

NOTE: No one will be permitted to visit without this
pass.
Please keep it in sight at all times and return it
to the information desk as you leave so that
others may visit the patient.

(over)

TWO VISITORS ONLY AT A TIME   **15 MINUTES PER VISIT**

GENERAL VISITING REGULATIONS

1. DO NOT VISIT IF YOU HAVE A COLD.

2. DO NOT SMOKE IN PATIENT'S ROOM.

3. DO NOT SIT ON PATIENT'S BED.

4. DO NOT BRING FOOD TO PATIENT.

5. LIMIT YOUR VISIT SO AS NOT TO TIRE THE
PATIENT AND ALSO GIVE OTHERS AN
OPPORTUNITY TO VISIT.

(over)

Figure 22. Sample visitor's pass. (*Courtesy of* St. Joseph's Hospital and
Medical Center, Paterson, New Jersey.)

SAINT BARNABAS MEDICAL CENTER

LIVINGSTON, N. J.

VISITOR'S
PASS NO. **035736**

THIS PASS SHOULD BE SURRENDERED WHEN LEAVING

SMOKING IN DESIGNATED AREAS ONLY
SPEED LIMIT 15 MPH BADGE NO.

VISITOR'S NAME	DATE / /
REPRESENTING COMPANY	PHONE NO.
COMPANY'S ADDRESS	
VEHICLE LICENSE NO.	STATE

PURPOSE OF VISIT

☐ SALES OR SERVICE ☐ DELIVERY ☐ PICKUP ☐ EMPLOYMENT

TO SEE:
1. _____ DEPT. _____

2. _____ DEPT. _____

3. _____ DEPT. _____

ARTICLES CARRIED IN BY VISITOR:

☐ HAND BAG ☐ PACKAGE ☐ OTHER
☐ BRIEF CASE ☐ NONE _____

X _____
SIGNATURE OF VISITOR

HAVE THIS PASS SIGNED BEFORE LEAVING EACH OFFICE YOU VISIT

VISITOR SEEN BY (INITIALS & TIME)

1.	2.		3.	
SIGNED IN BY:	TIME	SIGNED OUT BY		TIME

Figure 23. (*Courtesy of* St. Barnabas Medical Center, Livingston, New Jersey.)

(3) Return the pass to the main desk.

(4) Others may be waiting!

Visitor Workmen — Service Control

Not all hospital visitors are family and friends wishing to see patients. Some are salespeople, delivery people, repair workers, and others that have business to conduct within the hospital complex. These visitors should be instructed through posted signs at entrances to report to the information desk or a security check point where they can state their business and receive a pass. A visitor's log should be maintained whereby the visitor signs his name and organization representation, the time, and whom he is going to visit.

Upon signing the visitor's log, a pass will be issued to the visitor. This pass, along with a visitor's badge, will enable the visitor to conduct his business within the hospital complex. The visitor's pass must be countersigned by the authorized hospital representative being visited. Upon leaving the hospital, the pass must be surrendered at the same check point entered. The security officer will then note the visitor's departure time in the log.

SELECTED READINGS

Bastoni, Jeannie: The small company faces visitor control. *Industrial Security*, February 1970.

Holt, Kenneth M.: Security hostess aid hospital visitor control. *Hospital Topics*, July 1969.

Leydon, Joseph J.: Salesman's pass aids security and product selection. *Modern Hospital*, August 1968.

Lipper, C.: Good signs can help control visitor and staff traffic. *Modern Hospital*, July 1970.

MacDonald, Morgan B., Jr. and Brown, James K.: Company security practices. *The Conference Board Record*, IV (10): 40-47, October 1967.

Smith, Mack: Designing a visitor's pass system. *Hospital Topics*, 35, January 1970.

———: A successful hospital visitor's pass. *Security World*, 6(9):46, October 1969.

Chapter 14

PATIENTS' VALUABLES PROCEDURE

HOSPITALS are not in the business of safe-guarding money and valuables for patients. They are in the business of healing patients. Unfortunately, however, the hospital administration cannot ignore the safety of patients' money and valuables. To do so would be irresponsible. Any hospital that does not have a system for protecting the patients' valuables should develop a policy that can reduce the loss of patients' valuables.

The ideal situation for protecting the patients' valuables is to have a policy that requires valuables to be sent home with relatives and friends. Patients should be advised of this policy at the time of admission. They should also be advised that the hospital does not assume responsibility for cash and valuables retained by the patient. The policy of requiring valuables to be sent home, however, does not in itself solve the problem since it is not always practical nor desirable to do so. A procedure should be developed to protect the valuables retained in the hospital. This procedure should require that valuables and cash be deposited immediately with the business office in order to be protected. The use of a valuables envelope is strongly recommended.

Depositing Procedure At Admission

The admitting office should routinely inform the patient and/or relatives that valuables not immediately sent home must be deposited with the hospital for safekeeping. In the event the patient desires to have the hospital keep his valuables, admitting must complete a "Valuables Envelope" and promptly deliver it to the cashier. The receipt will be attached to the patient's medical record.

DIRECTIONS FOR COMPLETING VALUABLES ENVELOPE: All entries are to be made in ink. The amount of money and the name of valuables are to be listed on the envelope. The patient or his relatives will acknowledge by means of signature that the contents listed are correct and the signature will be witnessed by the appropriate hospital personnel. Signatures of acceptance by nursing, admitting, and business office personnel must be complete names — not initials.

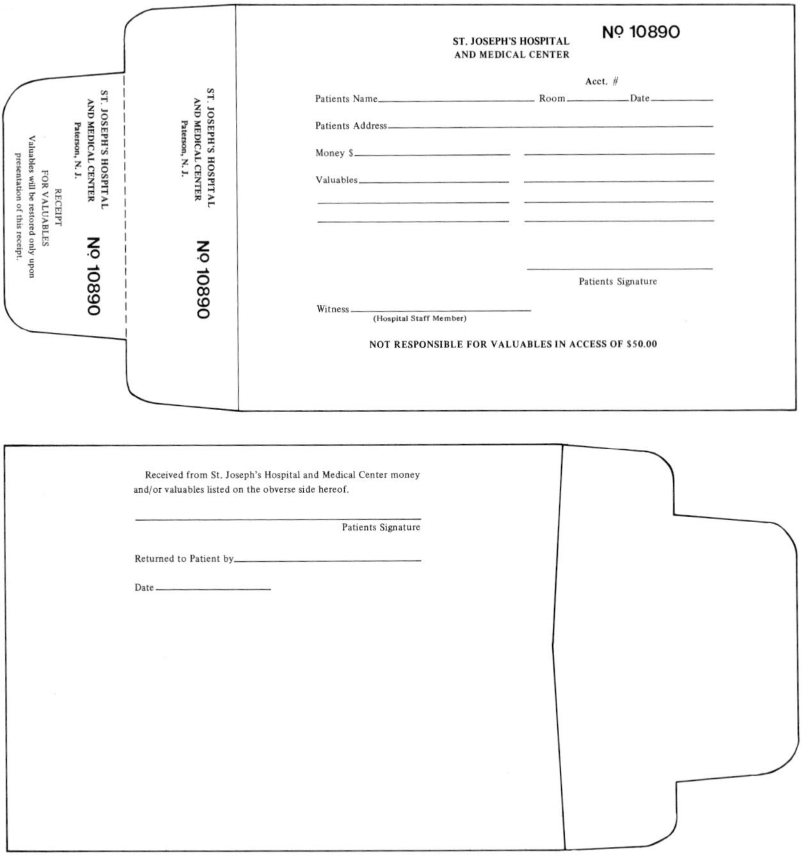

Figure 24.

AFTER HOURS ADMISSION OR EMERGENCY ROOM ADMISSIONS. If a patient wishes to have the hospital keep his valuables, a member of the nursing department will complete and seal a "Valuables Envelope" and deliver said valuables to the cashier's office where a receipt will be given by the cashier for attachment to the patient's chart. The envelope, together with its contents, will then be secured in the hospital safe. In the event the cashier's office is closed, e.g. on holidays, the envelope should be delivered to the out-patient business office. A receipt will be given to the representative from nursing. The valuables envelope, together with its contents, should be promptly deposited into the night depository box. Envelopes deposited during evening hours should be transported to the cashier's office on the following day as soon as it opens so all valuables will be stored at a central location.

Valuables Kept By Patients

A valuables drawer should be established at each nursing station for the purpose of *temporarily storing* minor jewelry items and a small amount of cash (maximum to be established by the hospital) for a period not to exceed *twenty-four hours,* for patients going to surgery, etc. The key and control of the valuables drawer is the responsibility of the nurse supervisor at each station and the drawer is to be kept locked at all times.

Withdrawal Procedure

At the time of discharge, the patient's cash and valuables retained by the hospital in his behalf will be released by the cashier subsequent to surrender of the proper receipt by the patient or his designate. The envelope with its corresponding receipt stapled to it will then be filed in the business office valuables file.

Valuables and/or money will be returned only upon presentation of the proper receipt. Under NO circumstances will an envelope seal be broken for an interim withdrawal and resealed. For partial withdrawals, the entire contents must be receipted by the depositor and a new envelope prepared for any remaining valuables requiring safe-keeping. The old envelope will be filed in the business office valuables file.

Release of Deceased Patient's Valuables

Valuables of a deceased patient, including patients dead on arrival, will be released to the next of kin or the funeral director subject to obtaining proper identification and signatures on the "Valuables Envelope Receipt." The envelope, together with its corresponding receipt, will then be filed within the business office valuables file.

SELECTED READINGS

Brown, John F.: Security spotlight, security management plant and property protection. *National Foreman's Institute*, No. 415, August 10, 1975. [Bureau of Business Practices, Waterford, Conn.]

Carlson, Gus: Theft prevention controls — A must for hospitals. *Hospital Topics*, July 1969.

Dailey, Edward J., Jr.: Security programs needed to insure patients and personnel safety. *Hospital Topics*, November 1968.

Horty, John F.: Patient security is a contractual obligation. *Modern Hospital*, *103* (No. 1):94, July 1964.

Chapter 15

INTEGRATED SECURITY SYSTEMS

T HE use of integrated security systems and supplemental electronic equipment in hospitals and health care institutions is becoming an essential security support system. It should be emphasized at the outset that integrated security systems that utilize closed circuit television and other electronic security devices are not intended to replace a viable security force; rather, these devices are intended to be of aid and assistance to the security force.

The determination to use or not to use supporting electronic security systems will be determined in large part by the size and location of the hospital complex, the unique and individual security needs of the hospital, and the financial considerations in purchasing and maintaining the equipment. These factors must be carefully weighed before any sizable investments are made. Serious shopping should take place. Various products should be compared against each other for durability, reliability, easy maintenance, and above all for effectiveness. An essential factor when considering the purchase of electronic security equipment is the technical advice and service that accompanies the product.

In order to understand how an integrated security system functions, one should understand the individual components that comprise the system. One of the basic components of an electronic security system, and often the heart of the system, is closed circuit television.

CLOSED CIRCUIT TELEVISION. Otherwise known by the initials CCTV, this system has improved considerably over the last ten years. Low light-level models are now sufficiently developed to transmit clear and vivid images from areas that are in either near total darkness or bright sunlight. A security officer at a central station can monitor as many as fifteen areas from one location. From this central location he can dispatch, as the need arises, security patrol officers to trouble spots.

The closed circuit television cameras can be augmented by the integration of video tape recorders, VTR, that can provide a permanent visual record on tape. The playback capability of the video tape recorder is its strongest selling point. This system reduces the need for constant visual monitoring by a security officer.

Some additional features of CCTV are the following:

- Cameras can be mounted on a pan or tilt device to move cameras horizontally and/or vertically.
- Cameras can be equipped with zoom lenses controlled by the monitoring security officer.
- Cameras can be concealed to monitor emotionally disturbed patients.
- Cameras can be equipped with dual lenses to provide two images on one monitor with different magnifications and different scenes.
- Cameras can be set up to perform either random or sequential monitoring of an area.

Utilizing Computers in the Integrated Security System

With the aid of a computer in the integated security system, the central monitoring station can be programed to:

- control life safety systems such as fire and smoke detection.
- activate warning signals and alarms relative to unlawful entry, sabotage, vandalism, and other disasters.
- switch lights on and off.
- test and reset sensing devices.
- monitor equipment malfunctions.
- admit or deny access to the hospital by opening and closing doors.
- provide permanent print-outs of employees granted admittance to the hospital, or selected areas such as the pharmacy, via magnetically coded identification card keys. The print-out could include the employee identification card

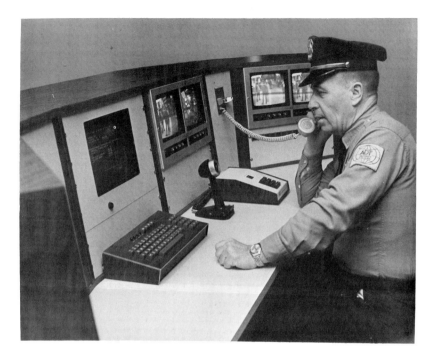

Figure 25. At the central monitoring station, a large security console includes CCTV screens for monitoring remote areas of the hospital. (*Courtesy of* ADT Security Systems.)

number, status level, date, time, and location.

Base Radio Station

Two way communication between the command post and the security patrol has become increasingly efficient through the use of a base radio station at the command post. Security officers are equipped with two-way radios that are compact, durable, and most dependable. The command post can dispatch roving security officers to trouble spots within minutes. The roving security officers can also keep in direct communication with the security command post and alert the command to any unusual happenings or request assistance as the need

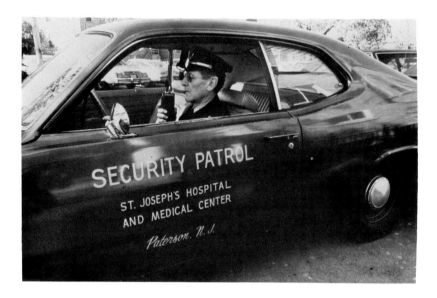

Figure 26. The roving security officer keeps in direct communication with the security command post.

arises.

Another frequently used audio transceiver is a pagemaster. This device, however, does not allow for immediate, direct two-way communication. It emits a tone signal to the receiver who then telephones his office or command post for further instructions. The pagemaster's compact size, the size of a cigarette package, and dependability have made it extremely popular within hospitals.

When all or part of the individual components discussed above are interfaced, along with a host of other optional electronic security equipment, the result is an integrated security system. Remember that an integral part of the integrated electronic security system is qualified security personnel. The system will only be as efficient as the personnel who monitor and respond to the equipment output.

A few final points to be considered before implementing an integrated security system:

•Review all cost factors including potential savings.

•Plan your system to meet your specific hospital needs, while allowing for possible future expansion of the system.

•Avoid hasty judgments and misapplication of equipment.

•Seek advice from those who have systems in operation.

SELECTED READINGS

Astor, Saul: Should management invest in electronic security? *Security World, 11* (1):30-33, January 1974.

CCTV has as yet only been lightly touched upon. *Security World, 5* (No. 3): March 1968.

Choosing security systems. *National Safety News, 90:*22, September 1964.

Cole, Richard B.: *The Application of Security Systems and Hardware.* Springfield, Thomas, 1970.

Desrosiers, A. L.: Security systems in hospitals. *Hospital Topics, 43:*51, March 1965; 51-54, April 1965.

Electronic sentinels can increase the security and reduce the payroll. *Modern Hospital,* 96-97, July 1968.

Eversull, Kennen: Automatic plant protection. *Factory,* December 1961.

———: Consideration in radio communications. *Security World, 5* (No. 9):31-44, October 1968.

———: Planning the communications center, part I. *Security World, 5* (No. 8):12-15, September 1968.

———: Planning the communications center, part II. *Security World, 5* (No. 11), December 1968.

Goldman, Elliot H.: Security and the technology of loss prevention. *Security World 9* (6):44-47, June 1972.

Leydon, Joseph J.: Salesman's pass aids security and product selection. *Modern Hospital, III:*54, August 1968.

Mahoney, Bill: Electronic eyes. *Law and Order, 9:* November, 1961.

———: Protecting life and property with TV. *Law and Order 12:* May 1964.

Miller, Floyd G.: Practical solutions to entrance security for large area, multiple buildings. *Security World,* II, (#9): 16-20, October 1974.

Nielson, George E.: Computerized access control. *Industrial Security,* October 1968.

Schilter, George R.: Hospital security systems — which is best for your hospital? *Financial Management,* 24-26, March 1969.

Special 10th anniversary reports on the future of electronics in security, A series of articles. *Security World, 10* (9):15-72, October 1973.

Weber, Thad L.: *Alarm Systems and Theft Prevention.* Los Angeles, Security World Publishing Co., Inc.

Chapter 16

ARREST, SEARCH, AND SEIZURE

THE whole realm of arrest, search, and sei-
zure is a complicated one. Entire criminal justice textbooks are
devoted to the subject. Many suspected criminals are not prose-
cuted by the courts due to technicalities in the arrest, search,
and seizure procedures used by law enforcement officers. The
authors, therefore, will not attempt to present a comprehensive
study of the subject but will highlight those aspects of the
subject area that private security officers should be familiar
with.

The Fourth Amendment to The United States Constitution

"The right of the people to be secure in their persons,
houses, papers, and effects, against unreasonable searches and
seizures, shall not be violated, and no Warrants shall be issued,
but upon probable cause, supported by Oath or affirmation,
and particularly describing the place to be searched, and the
persons or things to be seized."

The Fifth Amendment to The United States Constitution

"No person shall be held to answer for a capital, or otherwise
infamous crime, unless on a presentment or indictment of a
Grand Jury, except in cases arising in the land or naval forces,
or in the Militia, when in actual service in time of War or
public danger; nor shall any person be subject for the same
offense to be twice put in jeopardy of life or limb, nor shall be
compelled in any criminal case to be a witness against himself,
nor be deprived of life, liberty, or property, without due process
of law; nor shall private property be taken for public use,
without just compensation."

Both of these amendments in the Bill of Rights are important to the understanding of the subject of arrest, search, and seizure. It is these two amendments that clearly define the protection of an individual's privacy, which includes both his person and his property.

Arrest

As stated above, the fourth amendment prohibits "unreasonable seizures" of persons and property. Arrest, therefore, is a seizure of a person and is forbidden except on probable cause. Probable cause is defined as: A reasonable ground for suspicion, supported by circumstances sufficiently strong in themselves, to lead a cautious police officer to believe that the party is guilty of a crime.

If a private security officer, while on duty, were to stop and detain someone whom he merely suspected of stealing from the hospital and later the detained party is proven innocent of any wrongdoing, the security officer would then probably be sued in a court of law by the injured party for false arrest. Mere suspicion by a private security officer is not sufficient probable cause to detain a person for any length of time. That is not to say that a security officer should neglect to investigate suspicious acts of people within the hospital complex. Caution, common sense, and good judgment based on knowledge of the law should be your guide.

In some cases, security personnel are peace officers who are deputized with powers of arrest. In performing their duties, they would follow all of the prescribed procedures set down for a peace officer in initiating a lawful arrest. In complying with the fifth amendment to the Federal Constitution (no person "shall be compelled in a criminal case to be a witness against himself") a peace officer would inform an arrested subject of his rights. The Miranda decision requires that a person held in custody be informed of his right not to incriminate himself. Specifically, the Miranda warnings state:

(i) You have a right to remain silent and do not have to say anything at all.

(ii) Anything you say can and will be used against you in

court.

(iii) You have a right to talk to a lawyer of your own choice before we ask you any questions and also to have a lawyer here with you while we ask questions.

(iv) If you cannot afford to hire a lawyer, and you want one, we will see that you have a lawyer provided to you before we ask you any questions.

If a person is arrested by a peace officer and later found innocent of the charge against him, the peace officer would not be personally liable to a false arrest suit. The majority of hospital security officers, however, are not peace officers and only have arrest powers as a private person. If a security officer, as a private person, makes an arrest that does not hold up in court, he can be personally liable in a civil suit against him.

As a private person, a security officer may make an arrest when a crime has been committed or attempted in his presence. An arrest cannot be made by a security officer on hearsay evidence. By an arrest is meant the taking into custody a person, under real or assumed authority, with the purpose of holding that person to answer a criminal charge. If an arrest is made by a private security officer, the prisoner must be delivered to a peace officer immediately. To delay could make the arrest unlawful.

The hospital security officer is not in the business of arresting criminals. It has been stated countless times throughout this text that the officer's job is the protection of life and property. If the officer sees anything suspicious, he should call his chief and inform him of what is taking place. The police department should then be notified. When the police arrive, they will make an arrest based on the information given them, i.e. probable cause furnished by the security officer.

Search and Seizure

Prior to the Bill of Rights, the colonists were subjected to arbitrary searches by the British who had the authority under a "Writ of Assistance" to conduct general searches and seizures. Under this authority, the British officials could open any package and confiscate any item in the "Name of the King". The fourth amendment of the Bill of Rights corrected this wrong. The amendment guarantees the citizenry freedom from arbitrary and unlawful searches. Specifically, the amendment states "The right of the people to be secure in their persons, houses, papers and effects, against unreasonable searches and seizures" etc.

A search must, with few exceptions, be made under an authorized search warrant, issued only to police officers. It is not made available to private security officers. In order to obtain a warrant, a police officer goes to a Magistrate. The officer makes out an affidavit which contains the "probable cause" as to why he wants to search a particular place. The area to be searched must be specified in the affidavit for a search warrant. This warrant is good for a reasonable length of time, normally not to exceed ten days from the date of issue. Normally, a search warrant may be executed only in the daytime, unless specifically stated on the warrant.

Four Ways to Make a Search

A lawful search can be made in four ways.
1. With a validly issued search warrant.
2. Searches incidental to arrest.
3. Emergency searches of automobiles.
4. Voluntary consent of the individual who has knowledge of his right not to consent to a search.

The ideal and safest way to insure a valid search is for a police officer to obtain a search warrant prior to the search. Since hospital security officers do not have authorized peace powers, they cannot obtain search warrants nor should they be engaged in searches of individuals and their personal property. What then can a security officer do? A security officer is permitted to look into the bag of anyone entering the hospital or require bags to be checked at a security location. If a person refuses, the officer has the right to refuse entry into the hospital. If a security officer sees someone walking out with hospital property, he can hold the person until the police arrive. The security officer, however, must make a complaint before the police can make an arrest. If the security officer cannot detain the person leaving with hospital property he should attempt to supply the police with an accurate report that includes a description of the suspect, a description of the valuables taken, and the direction and transportation used by the suspect. The police will then take over the investigation. The security department, in the above situation, should then limit their involvement to supplying the police with any additional information that may help solve the case.

SELECTED READINGS·

Cohen, Stanley: *A Law Enforcement Guide to United States Supreme Court Decisions.* Springfield, Thomas, 1972.

Davis, Rev D.: *Federal Searches and Seizures.* Springfield, Thomas, 1964.

United States Department of Justice *Handbook on The Law of Search and Seizure.* Superintendent of Documents, United States Government Printing Office, Washington, D. C., January 1967.

The Police Administration and Public Safety College of Social Science, Michigan State University: *Law and Order Training for Civil Defense Emergency, Student Manual* (Part B). East Lansing, Mich St U Pr, August 1965.

Schwartz, Louis B. and Goldstein, Stephen R.: *Law Enforcement Handbook For Police.* St. Paul, West Publishing Co., 1970.

Sutton, John F., Jr.: Authority person not an officer to arrest for a misdemeanor. *Security World,* 2 (No. 7): October 1965.

———: Law in the security world, false imprisonment. *Security World,* 2, (No. 6): September 1965.

———: Law in the security world: The authority of a person not an officer to arrest for a misdemeanor. *Security World,* 2 (No. 7): October 1965.

Van De Kamp, John K.: Search and seizure, part I. *Security World,* 5 (No. 1): January 1968.

———: Search and seizure, part II. *Security World,* 5 (No. 2): February 1968.

Chapter 17

WRITTEN REPORTS

The Necessity for Reports

THE primary purpose of written reports is to provide the hospital security organization with a permanent record of information. It is for this reason that reports are filled out, dated, and filed. Thus, reports keep the administrative officers abreast of current and past events while serving as a basis for future administrative decisions.

Reports furnish the necessary information to security administrative officers so that they can effectively coordinate the planning and supervision of the department's activities. With information gathered on who is doing what, how, when, and where it is being done, and what action is being taken, the command officers may then effectively direct the activities of the department. For example, reports can indicate that a heavier patrol is needed in a certain area at a certain time, or that firefighting equipment is faulty and needs replacement.

A security officer becomes the eyes and ears of the hospital. It is his job function to report unusual incidents that occur in the hospital complex, e.g. vandals, drunks, fist fights, unauthorized intruders. It is also the security officer's duty to report unsafe conditions within the hospital complex, such as faulty wiring, closed sprinkler valves, electrical equipment left running, broken steps and windows, leaky faucets, and the like. Further, the security officer is responsible for protecting the property of the hospital and all of its inhabitants. Stolen articles, whether from the hospital pharmacy, the hospital laundry, the hospital kitchen, or from a patient's room, are incidents that are to be directed to the security department. It is the security department's responsibility to file a report in order to provide the basis for an investigation and/or a permanent record for a follow-up procedure.

All of the above situations require a written report. It is the security officer's duty to generate these reports. It is usually impractical for a security officer to follow through on an incident from beginning to end. The reports left by the originating officer furnish the information necessary for other officers to carry the case through to a successful conclusion.

The reasons for security reports might be summarized as follows:

1. To provide a permanent record of information.
2. To communicate information.
3. To enable security administrative officers to evaluate whether the information is being properly handled.
4. To keep administrative officers abreast of current events.
5. To serve as a basis for administrative decisions.
6. To provide, when necessary, a basis for the continuation of an investigation by others.
7. To serve as a basis for the dissemination of information to the police and the courts in cases resulting in litigation.

Reports are the foundation upon which modern security work is built. Clear, concise, and accurate reports should be the objective of each and every security officer. An important part of writing accurate reports is the ability to take good field notes. When actually completing the report, not all details can be remembered. If you take good notes, immediately or shortly thereafter, they will provide the basis for your report. The notebook and pen, therefore, are very important tools in security work. A security officer should never leave the scene until he is certain that all pertinent information necessary to write an adequate report has been documented.

The report must always be factual. Record facts as they are obtained. Valuable time and effort can be lost if the report does not contain the right information.

Five important questions to be asked in filling out any report are: who, what, where, when, and how? To assist the security officer in understanding the above five important questions, the following can be asked about each.

WHO? Who originated the report to the security department?

Who is the victim? Who is the alleged perpetrator(s)? Who witnessed the incident? Who discovered the incident? Who can be contacted later for additional information? List names, addresses, telephone numbers, descriptions where needed.

WHAT? What happened? What was taken? Describe in detail exactly what took place. What was damaged? What was left unattended? (e.g. an open elevator shaft) What evidence was left at the scene? What action was taken by the security officer in charge? What further action needs to be taken? What were the conditions of the scene, such as distances, lighting, noises, etc.? What were the physical and emotional state of the witnesses?

WHERE? Where did the incident take place? Where was the suspect sighted? Where was the witness in relation to the incident? Where was the property before it was stolen?

WHEN? When did the incident occur — try to pinpoint the exact time of day? When was the incident reported to the security department — be exact on the time? When did the security officer arrive at the scene of the incident? When was the suspect sighted by witnesses?

How? How did the incident occur? How did the intruder enter the premises? How did the thief leave the hospital? How was the theft discovered? How were the police notified?

An additional question could be asked — "Why did it happen?" What incidents led to the happening that this report describes? This should include the events immediately preceding the offense.

After you have made out a report ask yourself the following questions:

1. Is it complete? Does it answer the questions who, what, where, when, how, and why?
2. Is it accurate and specific? It must be based on facts.
3. Is it easy to understand?
4. Is it concise? Does it contain extra words that are not necessary or important?
5. Is it grammatically correct?

Reports all have value if they are used correctly. Making

investigations is very important. The investigator must know how to get information from people and how to evaluate it. Evidence is that which tends to prove or disprove any matter.

Kinds of Evidence

There are four kinds of evidence:

1. Direct — based on personal knowledge.
2. Circumstantial — logical, but no one can really prove the way it happened.
3. Real — speaks for itself and requires no explanation, such as photographs, maps, X-rays.

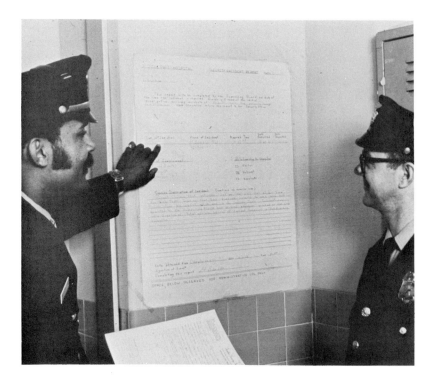

Figure 27. Security officers review posted procedures necessary for completing an incident report. (*Courtesy of* Frontier Security, Inc.)

4. Hearsay — information relayed from one person to another or rumor.

Proof is testimony or convincing evidence. Without evidence there is no proof.

Everybody uses a different system in making out reports, but basically every system should answer the questions mentioned above. All reports must be properly dated and signed by the person making out the report. Reports should contain no opinions, only facts. Reports are often considered the best gauge of the pride, interest, abilities, and knowledge of the person making the report. A deep personal satisfaction can be derived from submitting comprehensive reports.

When asked to write a report, do the best job possible. Supervisors read them, administrators often see them, and the hospital director also reads them.

APPENDIX
Security Officers Log

SECURITY OFFICERS LOG

POST # _____

DUTY TOUR _____   NAME _____
DATE   TOUR

TIME	EVENT	ACTION TAKEN
	SIGNATURE	PAGE _____ of _____ PAGES

SE-2

SECURITY INCIDENT REPORT REJECT SLIP

TO:

FROM:

- -

REASON REPORT WAS REJECTED

Incomplete Information ( )

Illegible Writing ( )

- -

NEED ADDITIONAL INFORMATION CONCERNING

Date   ( )   Place   ( )

Time   ( )   Incident ( )

Other ( )

Comments: _____

_____

- -

INSTRUCTIONS

Please complete as indicated and return to_____Security Department.

- -

Courtesy of Saint Joseph's Hospital and Medical Center.

Security Incident Report

DATE_____

INSTRUCTIONS: This report is to be completed by the supervising guard on duty at the time the incident is reported. Guards will conduct the initial investigation involving incidents of: *Assault, Theft, Fire, Property Damage, Vandalism* and *Auto Accidents.* Upon completion, return this report to the Security Office.

Type of Incident	Place of Incident	Approx. Time	date occurred	date reported

Name of Complainant   *Relationship to Hospital*
( ) Visitor ( ) Patient ( ) Employee

Concise Description of Incident (Continue on reverse side if necessary)

_____

_____

_____

_____

_____

_____

_____

_____

_____

Info. obtained from:_____ date_____ time_____

Signature of guard completing report_____

SPACE BELOW RESERVED FOR ADMINISTRATIVE USE ONLY . . . .

Courtesy of St. Joseph's Hospital and Medical Center.

Missing Property

Date:_____ Time:_____

Loss reported by:	( ) employee ( ) visitor ( ) patient
Owner of property:	( ) employee ( ) visitor ( ) patient

Address: City:

State: Department:

Phone: extension Officer making report:

Police ( ) yes If no
called: ( ) no explain:

Name of police officer:	Badge number:

Who called Police: Permission to call by:

Loss in Dept.
Dept. Head called: Time

Investigation of Loss

Building where loss occurred: Floor: Unit or room:

Grounds Area: Parking stall: Light post:

Description of property in full:

Estimated value: ( ) old If old
( ) new how old; Color:

Serial number: Identification Marks:

Where was item when last seen or used:

Who saw or used item: Time item last seen or used:

Date last seen or used: Where was item kept:

→

Time loss	( ) am	Time loss		( ) am	Time loss
Discovered:	( ) pm	Reported:		( ) pm	between:

Date loss	Date loss	Days
discovered:	reported	between:

Type of control
system used

Who was in charge of
system at time of loss:

Are keys	( ) yes	If yes how are
used in system:( ) no		they controled:

(over)

Missing Property - reverse

Who was responsible
for key control system:

Is a key control   ( ) yes   Where is
box used in system: ( ) no   it located:

Were keys   ( ) yes   If yes
checked out: ( ) no   by whom:

How is system
checked:

Who checked it
last and when: Date: Time:

Are there other   ( ) yes   Who has
keys: ( ) no   them:

Notes or remarks:

Doors	Windows:	Lockers:
( ) Locked	( ) Locked	( ) Locked
( ) Unlocked	( ) Unlocked	( ) Unlocked
( ) Lock forced	( ) Lock forced	( ) Lock forced
( ) Key used	( ) Glass broken	( ) Door forced
( ) Glass broken		

Automobile

Make: Year: Color:

License: State: Serial
                                                       number

Body: 2 Door ( )
                                           4 Door ( )

Badge No._____   Patrolman Signature X _____

Alarm Sound ( ) yes ( ) no

Courtesy of Holy Name Hospital Teaneck, New Jersey.

Offense Reporting Form

| Courtesy: Saint Barnabas Medical Center
Livingston, N. J. | | | | | | **SECURITY DEPARTMENT** | |

OFFENSE CATEGORY	Date-Time Received	Day of Wk.	Date Mo. Day Yr.	Time AM. PM.	Investigation No.

	Forced entry	Complainants Name		Home Phone

	Pers. Prop.	Address		Business Phone
	Med. Cntr. Prop.			
Theft	Coin Machine			
	Auto	Status		
	Narcotics	☐ Patient ☐ Visitor ☐ Employee ☐ Other (Specify)		
Robbery				
Assault		DATE-TIME OF OFFENSE	Day of wk.	Date Mo. Day Year	Time AM. PM.
Rape					
Manslaughter					
Disturbance		Place		Weapon Used
Vandalism				
Traffic		Trademark		

Other
(Specify)

Victims Name		Address

Sex ☐ M ☐ F	Age	Race	Status ☐ Patient ☐ Visitor ☐ Employee ☐ Other (specify)

Medical Treatment ☐ Yes (Explain) ☐ No	Description of Lost Property	Value

DESCRIPTION OF OFFENDER(S)

No. 1	Sex ☐M ☐F	Race	Height	Build	Eyes	Hair	Glasses ☐Yes ☐No	Complexion
	Marks				Age	Hat	Coat	Shirt

No. 2	Sex ☐M ☐F	Race	Height	Build	Eyes	Hair	Glasses ☐Yes ☐No	Complexion
	Marks				Age	Hat	Coat	Shirt

Witness' Name	Address	Telephone
Witness' Name	Address	Telephone

LAW ENFORCEMENT AGENCY NOTIFIED	TIME	PERSON
	A.M. P.M.	
	A.M. P.M.	

Name of Person Arrested	Address
Name of Person Arrested	Address

CHARGES

Was Physical Force Used
☐ Yes   ☐ No

Signature of Reporting Officer Date	For Security Office Use Only Approved _____ Date Name Card Completed_____

(over)

Narrative — be specific in writing of this report. Be sure to use the guidelines, "who", "what", "when", "why", "where", "how". Describe offense in detail. Include initial statements uttered by victim, witnesses and suspects. Example: In car theft, what was victim's response to direct question, "was car locked?"? Describe scene of offense and contributory conditions such as poor lighting, extreme isolation, etc. List evidence found at scene and all other relevant information such as sobriety of victim, witnesses and suspects. Safeguard report for reference.

FOR SECURITY DEPARTMENT USE ONLY

This offense is declared:

Unfounded ☐
Cleared by arrest ☐
Exceptionally cleared ☐
Inactive (not cleared) ☐

Signed_____ Date_____
　　　　　　　　Security Director

Courtesy: Saint Barnabas Medical Center, Livingston, N. J.

Supplementary Offense Report

OFFENSE CATEGORY   INVESTIGATION NO.

COMPLAINANT   (LAST NAME)   (MIDDLE NAME)   (FIRST NAME)

ADDRESS

ADDITIONAL DETAILS OF OFFENSE, PROGRESS, OR INVESTIGATION, ETC.

THIS OFFENSE IS DECLARED:

Unfounded   ( )   Signed _____ Date _____
Cleared by Arrest   ( )   Investigating Officer
Exceptionally Cleared ( )   Signed _____ Date _____
Inactive (not cleared) ( )   Security Director

THIS FORM IS USED BY OFFICER ASSIGNED TO A CASE TO REPORT PRO-
GRESS AFTER THREE AND SEVEN DAYS AND WEEKLY THEREAFTER. ALSO
TO REPORT SIGNIFICANT DEVELOPMENTS.

Courtesy of Saint Barnabas Medical Center, Livingston, New Jersey.

Lost and Found

Location Where Found: _____

Found By _____ Title _____

Received By: _____ Badge No. _____

Items: 1. _____

2. _____

3. _____

4. _____

5. _____

Name _____

Address _____

Town _____ State _____

Tel. _____ Employee _____ Dept. _____

Missing Items (Items claimed missing) _____

_____

Signature
All Found In Order? Yes ( ) No ( )   of Owner _____

How Identification Was Made _____

_____

Released By _____ Badge No. _____

(use reverse side if additional space is required)

Receipt

Received From_____Date _____

Items_____

_____

_____

Officers
Signature_____Badge No._____

Courtesy of Holy Name Hospital, Teaneck, New Jersey.

Missing Person

Time of Report:_____ Date of Report:_____ Time Cancelled:_____

Reported By:_____ Floor or Unit: _____

Supervisor Called: _____ Ext. _____

Name:_____ Room:_____ Bed: _____

Home Address:_____ Town: _____

Tel. #_____ Police Called: _____

Description of Person:

Height:_____ Weight:_____ Hair:_____ Age:_____ Sex:_____

Color:_____ Eyeglasses:_____ Scars or Marks: _____

Characteristics: _____

Suit or Dress:_____ Coat: _____

Pants or Skirt:_____ Shirt: _____

Sweater:_____ Hat:_____ Tie:_____ Shoes: _____

Other Clothing or Items: _____

Possible Whereabouts: _____

In Company of:_____

Last Seen:_____ Time: _____

Reason For Leaving: _____

Note:_____

_____

_____

Buildings Checked:_____ Grounds Checked:_____ Time:_____

Officer & Shield #_____

Officer In Charge:_____

Courtesy of Holy Name Hospital, Teaneck, New Jersey.

Report of Motor Vehicle Accident	Exact Date of Accident	Time AM PM	Day of Week	Guard Making Report (Signature)		
Light Conditions ☐ Light ☐ Dawn ☐ Dusk ☐ Dark	Weather ☐ Clear ☐ Snow ☐ Rain ☐ Fog	No. Vehicles Involved	Date Reported	Time	Reported By	

Vehicle #1	Vehicle #2
Operator's Name (Print)	Operator's Name (Print)
Address (Street and Number)	Address (Street and Number)
City State	City State
If H.N.H. Employed No. Dept. Sex	If H.N.H. Employed No. Dept. Sex
Driver's License No. ☐ Operator ☐ Chauffeur	Driver's License No. ☐ Operator ☐ Chauffeur
Owner's Name (Print)	Owner's Name (Print)
Address (Street and Number)	Address (Street and Number)
City State	City State
Year and Make of Vehicle	Year and Make of Vehicle
Car License No.	Car License No.
Describe Damage to Vehicle	Describe Damage to Vehicle

Names and Addresses of Persons in Vehicle #1	Names and Addresses of Persons in Vehicle #2
Name (Print)	Name (Print)
Address	Address
If H.N.H Employed No. Dept. Sex	If H.N.H. Employed No. Dept. Sex
Name (Print)	Name (Print)
Address	Address
If H.N.H. Employed No. Dept. Sex	If H.N.H. Employed No. Dept. Sex
Witnesses	Witnesses
Name (Print)	Name (Print)
Address	Address
If H.N.H. Employed No. Dept. Sex	If H.N.H. Employed No. Dept. Sex
Name (Print)	Name (Print)
Address	Address
If H.N.H. Employed No. Dept. Sex	If H.N.H. Employed No. Dept. Sex
Damage to Property Other Than Vehicle	Damage to Property Other Than Vehicle

Courtesy: Holy Name Hospital, Teaneck, N. J.   (over)

Describe bodily injury, if any, to persons involved

THIS PART FOR GUARD'S USE ONLY

Did local or state police make a report of this accident?

Driver's statement of how accident occurred in car #1

Driver's statement of how accident occurred in car #2

Condition of road at time of accident

1. ☐ Dry 2. ☐ Muddy 3. ☐ Snow 4. ☐ Wet 5. ☐ Icy

Type of road

1. ☐ Concrete 2. ☐ Black Top 3. ☐ Brick or Block 4. ☐ Dirt or Sand 5. ☐ Other

If traffic signals, which way were they set?

Description of accident by guard (if witness) or if not, by witness

Show how accident occurred by drawing diagram. To show path of vehicle before accident use solid line: after accident use dotted line: number each vehicle: show direction by arrow: show pedestrian by P; show railroad by ++++++; indicate north.

Disposition:

Signature of Sergeant

Courtesy: Holy Name Hospital, Teaneck, N. J.

SECURITY DEPARTMENT

MONTHLY TIME REPORT

NAME:_____ MONTH OF:_____

JOB TITLE:_____ FROM:_____TO:_____

REGULAR/PART-TIME:_____

DATE	SHIFT WORKED	REG. HOURS.	HRS. O.T. SPEC. DTY.	HRS. OFF ILLNESS	HRS. OFF VACATION	HRS. OFF HOLIDAY	OTHER (EXPLAIN)
1							
2							
3							
4							
5							
6							
7							
8							
9							
10							
11							
12							
13							
14							
15							
16							
17							
18							
19							
20							
21							
22							
23							
24							
25							
26							
27							
28							
29							
30							
31							

Certification: I certify to the accuracy and validity of recorded entries on this time sheet.

Signature:_____

Source: Muhlenburg Hospital.

Hospital Safety Report

TO: Plant Engineer

FROM: Director of Security

SUBJECT: Request for Repair or Removal of Physical Safety Hazards

LOCATION: _____

REASON FOR REQUEST: *(Explain in detail)*

_____

_____

_____

_____   _____

Signature of Reporting Officer   Signature of Director of Security

----

Disposition of Request

TO: Director of Security

FROM: Plant Engineer

SUBJECT: Safety Repair

Action Taken: _____

_____

No Action Taken — Reason: _____

_____

_____

Signature of Plant Engineer

SELECTED READINGS

A Guide to Security Investigations. The American Society For Industrial Security, Washington, D. C., 1970, 91 pgs.

Erhardt, John E.: *Investigation,* a paper presented at the Fifth Annual Institute For Hospital Security Guards, Greater New York Hospital Association, New York, 1971.

Gammage, Allen Z.: *Basic Police Report Writing.* Springfield, Thomas, 1974.

The Police Administration and Public Safety College of Social Science, Michigan State University: *Law and Order Training for Civil Defense Emergency, Student Manual* (Part B). East Lansing, Mich St U Pr, August 1965.

Love, Robert C.: The security officer's notebook. *Law and Order, 9,* January-April 1961.

Report Writing. Santa Cruz, Davis Publishing Co., 1971.

Section III

Hospital Safety

Chapter 18

FIRE PREVENTION AND CONTROL

THE primary responsibility of a hospital security officer is the protection of life and property. Fire prevention and control, therefore, are an integral part of a security officer's duties. Since fire threatens both life and property, the security officer must be thoroughly schooled in fire prevention, detection, control, extinguishment and evacuation. Moreover, his responsibility is carried even further to include staff training. The security department, in close cooperation with the local municipal fire department, should constantly train and retrain the entire hospital staff on emergency hospital fire safety.

Every hospital should have a well-organized fire safety plan. This plan should be based on a thorough knowledge of the hospital. The fire emergency plan should be closely coordinated by a predetermined method of procedure. A detailed "Hospital Fire Emergency Plan" is contained in this chapter.

Fire prevention in a hospital is every employee's concern. The security department, because of its responsibility to protect lives and property, must be extremely conscious of unsafe or hazardous conditions. They are in a natural position, through their patrol functions, to spot potential fire hazards. When they do uncover a potential fire hazard, they should take corrective action, where possible, and then fill out a report, for permanent record, of the incident. Appropriate copies should be sent to the department head where the hazard was identified, as well as to the maintenance engineer or safety director, so that malfunctions requiring technical knowledge can be corrected.

A typical fire hazard malfunction could be a faulty electrical system producing sparks. The security report would indicate the location of the faulty electrical system, the time, the day, and a description of the hazard. The security officer would see to it that this hazard was disconnected from use before leaving the scene. The report submitted to the maintenance engineer would have space available for him to indicate when and how the hazard was corrected. The report should then be returned to the security office and kept on permanent file.

Typical Hazards

Electrical Supply: Overloaded circuit containing too many machines, appliances, or lighting fixtures on a circuit.

Exposed electrical cords: Frayed wiring where the protective, insulated coating is worn exposing the wire.

Unattended Appliances: Machines, hot plates, coffee makers, etc. left on, especially overnight, can be very dangerous.

Unattended Open Flames: In kitchens, labs, etc.

Flammable Liquids: Gasoline and solvents that are uncapped or are not in "safety cans" (without seams) are extremely dangerous.

Oxygen Bottles: When not in use, should be properly capped. They should be stored in a special room, chained or racked so as not to tip. These bottles should be moved only on carts, properly chained.

Waste Storage: Waste material stored in stairwells or corridors should be removed. If exposed to fire, it will rapidly ignite and spread fire and toxic smoke upward in the open stairwell.

No Smoking Violations: Smoking should be confined to designated areas. Smoking is not permitted in clinics, laboratories, operating rooms, post operation rooms, oxygen storage areas, or other areas where volatiles are used.

Grease Buildup: Kitchen ventilation hoods should be free of grease buildup.

Spontaneous Ignition: Proper elimination of lint in the laundry and storage areas is essential. Linen and lint buildup may produce spontaneous combustion in hot, humid weather.

Cluttered Stairwells and Corridors: Stairwells and corridors must be kept free of obstacles. In case of fire, cluttered exits will reduce the efficiency of a speedy egress.

Faulty Fire Extinguishers: Broken nozzles, partially used extinguishers, etc., will hamper the control of a fire. An extinguisher with broken tags, missing tags, etc. should be reported and replaced.

Exit Signs: Missing or broken exit signs, especially illuminated exit signs, should be repaired or replaced.

Defective Fluorescent Light Ballasts: A defective fluorescent light ballast will usually produce a burnt odor and smoke. The light switch, where possible, should be shut off to break the current.

FIRE SAFETY EVACUATION PLAN

The essence of fire prevention consists of measures to elimi-

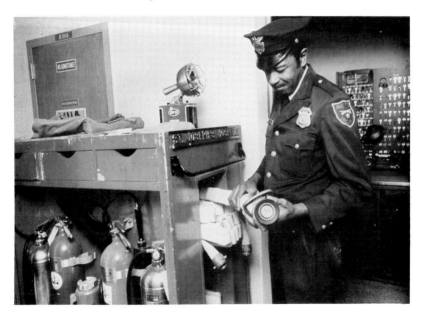

Figure 28. Security officer performs routine inspection of fire fighting equipment. (*Courtesy of* Frontier Security, Inc.)

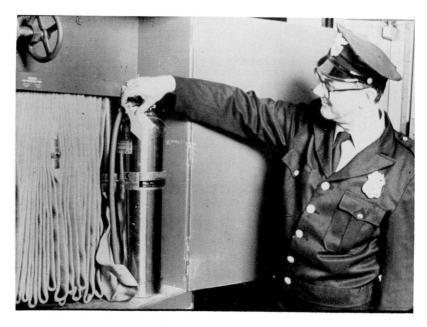

Figure 29. Security officer inspects fire extinguisher tags as part of the routine fire prevention inspection. Extinguishers with broken or missing tags should be reported and replaced. (*Courtesy of* Frontier Security, Inc.)

nate (or at least minimize the likelihood of) any condition suitable for combustion. Overall life safety involves much more, for long experience tells us that preventive measures cannot guard against every possibility. Consequently, a safety program must be predicated on the assumption that a fire may start in spite of all prevention efforts. Such a program must foresee all reasonable means of coping with fire and insuring against danger to life — by detecting fire's presence, by promptly sounding an alarm, and by effecting swift evacuation of the threatened premises, as well as by combating the fire, controlling its harmful emissions, and guarding against accidents and panic.

The life hazards arise from the products and immediate effects of fire and from the psychological impact of fire itself. Anyone near a fire is aware of heat, flame, light, and, usually, an odor or smoke. They may not be aware of various gases resulting from fire, nor of the fact that the oxygen supply is being depleted.

All these conditions may be contributors to the toll of human life — smoke by blinding, choking, and irritating; certain gases by poisoning; heat by searing and deep burning, often in unperceived ways, and, over and above the physical effects, the very presence of fire may lead to panic.

Once a fire has started, life safety demands the quickest possible sequence of detection, alarm, and evacuation, aided, in many instances, by measures to keep the fire in check at least until escape has been effected. A key point is that safety facilities and devices are effective only when integrated into an overall plan.

For the third and most vital step in life safety, namely, evacuation of the burning building, the normal means of departure may be supplemented by special routes; simultaneously, control measures and devices may be employed to keep the fire at bay and so lengthen the available escape time.

The evacuation route consists of the entire path from anywhere in the building to a safe point outside. Prudence dictates that at least two routes, normal or an alternate, be provided.

The normal pathways are those used in the daily movement of persons into and out of the building and from one activity to another. These generally comprise the doorways from each individual room or other interior rooms into corridors, along stairways, and through exits to the outside.

With lethal fires possible in any building, hazards of human error and faulty judgment must be reduced to a minimum. Every effort should be made to insure positive action and reactions to prevent fire as well as to insure safe evacuation if fire occurs.

Occupants of a building can help protect themselves and others from the consequences of fire by recognizing hazards that may be created by themselves or other, and knowing what to do in the event of fire.

Studies in the behavior of people show that knowledge and

training are essential in producing "right" responses. Many fire disasters could have been avoided had people been informed of the consequences of ill-considered (or unconsidered) behavior and had they been ready and willing to assume proper responsibilities.

Panic, for example, is likeliest to ensue when people feel themselves helpless or cut off from escape, do not know the way out, are not sure there is time to escape, or are not convinced that the escape route will be safe. It can arise from lack of knowledge about escape routes, or from lack of an alternate to a normal route which is (or is believed to be) blocked. Being prepared for an emergency requires that needed information be gathered, plans mapped, knowledge imparted, and training provided for all.

Devising effective evacuation plans differs sharply from scheduling normal movements of the occupants because there is no leeway for delay. Plans must take into account that someone should sound the alarm (even if the detection and alarm system is automatic), where people are likely to be when the alarm sounds, and what pattern of authority will exist for organized action.

Insofar as possible, clear lines of authority and responsibility should be established for each situation anticipated. Of particular importance will be the roles of the security director and the chief administrator, who are in a natural position to assume active leadership. The success of any plan will reflect their understanding of their responsibilities and their thoroughness in executing them. The following should be considered as the detailed evacuation plan is prepared:

- •Specific exit drill procedures should be prepared with floor plans and a copy of the procedure distributed to each member of the staff.
- •Staff meetings should be held during the year for instruction in the purposes and procedures of each drill, review of plans, and training new members while renewing the awareness of the rest.
- •Fire drills should be held at different times and under dif-

ferent conditions.
- Some drills should be conducted with some stairways and exits blocked.
- Provision should be made for evacuation of crippled or other wise incapacitated person.
- A different member of the staff should be called upon to sound the alarm each time to emphasize the importance of every member knowing where the alarm stations are located and how the alarm is operated and to help eliminate any psychological block a member may have against initiating an alarm.
- The alarm system should not be used for any purpose other than fire exit drill or actual fire alarm.
- The responsibility for prompt notification of the fire department should be assigned to persons who can assume it without delay.
- Cooperation should exist with fire department officials by calling drills in their presence or by advising them in advance of planned drills.
- Everyone should react immediately to an alarm. No one should stop for wraps or valuables. An alarm, once given, is never countermanded.
- "No Talking" regulations should be enforced during evacuation, to insure proper control at all times and to let everyone hear verbal orders.
- Attendance should be taken and the names of any persons unaccounted for should be reported to the chief administrator or person in charge.
- A report of each drill shall be prepared and kept on record. Pertinent details regarding evacuation should be recorded, such as the time taken to empty the building and recommendations for needed plan changes. (See "Fire Report" in chapter Appendix.)

Fire exit drills have three principal purposes: to insure rapid and safe evacuation during a real fire; to disclose unforeseen plan errors; and to reveal unreliable emergency behavior on the part of participants.

Each drill should be conducted as if there were a real fire. In priority of emergency actions, it should be made clear that sounding the alarm and starting people out of the building are most important.

It is a known fact that safety to life from fire in institutional buildings requires that the administrator and the staff give attention to and take adequate measures to meet their responsibility in all details affecting the fire safety of patients, which is often lost sight of where the needs for medical attention and care of patients absorb the attention of those in charge. It must be emphasized that the protection of the sick and helpless against loss of life by smoke or fire is a responsibility of importance comparable to that of medical attention.

The number of casualties, the amount of property damage, and the degree of panic reaction in the event of an emergency can be greatly reduced by the adoption of prescribed safety procedures and taking precautionary steps ahead of time. Planning and training directed toward the control of panic and hysteria, prompt attention to incipient fires and provision of first aid and rescue services are of primary importance to the hospital. A well-organized hospital security force can be the nucleus to provide the proper training in this area, via constant lectures, demonstrations, and fire drill practices.

The personnel should receive instructions in the use of first aid and fire extinguishment equipment. They should also be given instructions on emergency removal and various "carries" employed to evacuate the patients at the institution.

The purpose of fire exit drills is to insure the efficient and safe use of the exit facilities available. Proper drills insure orderly, controlled exit and prevent panic, (which has been responsible for the greater part of the loss of life in our major fire disasters). Order and control are the primary purposes of any fire drill. Speed of operations, while desirable, is not in itself an object and should be secondary to the maintenance of proper order and discipline.

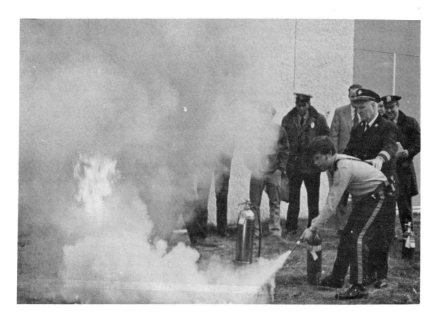

Figure 30. Security officers receive instruction by the local fire department on the proper procedures to follow in extinguishing a fire. (*Courtesy of* Jersey City State College.)

PREPLANNING FOR AN EMERGENCY

The words "Emergency Dr. Red" should be used over the intercommunication system to alert the security staff, institutional nurses, and other personnel in the event of fire.

Many times, the words "Fire Drill" set up a form of panic among the patients, causing undue work for the institutional staff. Since occupancies comprise, in large part, varied degrees of physical disability, removal of patients to the outside, or even disturbance of the patients by moving, is inexpedient or impractical in many cases, except as a last resort.

In order to set up a plan whereby only the staff personnel will know of a fire or a fire drill, the following terms will be used. "Dr. Red is visiting the institution" would mean that a fire drill is in progress. The term "Emergency Dr. Red" is used for the purpose of alerting the staff for a possible rapid evacuation of the building or the horizontal movement of patients from one area to a safer area behind properly maintained fire doors and fire wall separations. Fire is always unexpected, for this reason, drills are held when not expected. If a drill is always held in the same way at the same time, it loses much of its value; when, for some reason in an actual fire, it is not possible to follow the routine of the fire exit drill to which the occupants have become accustomed, confusion and panic may ensue. Fire exit drills are designed to familarize the occupants and the staff with all available means of egress, particularly fire escape stairs and other emergency exits that are not habitually used during the occupancy by the patients.

In order to secure proper order and control, it is essential that responsible persons competent to exercise leadership and carefully schooled in what to do in case of a fire emergency be on each floor to cope with any situation which may arise.

Fire fighting should always be made secondary to life safety. Special emphasis should be placed on not obstructing fire doors and lines of exit with fire hose until all patients are out of danger.

In most cases, fire and exit drills, as ordinarily practiced in other occupancies, cannot be conducted in institutions housing the sick and infirm.

Fundamentally, superior construction, early discovery and extinguishment of incipient fire, and prompt notification must be relied upon to reduce the occasion for evacuation in buildings of this class to a minimum.

Due to the generally low ratio of attendants to patients, no regular or constant designation of those responding to a fire alarm can be made. The person discovering a fire should immediately send an alarm from the nearest fire alarm box with the least disturbance and commotion and see that all doors adjacent to the fire are closed. He should advise another staff member of the location of the fire, who should confirm the

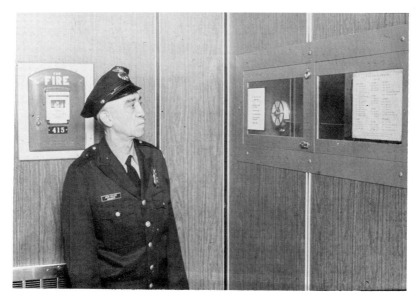

Figure 31. Security officer inspects posted safety instructions. (*Courtesy of Frontier Security, Inc.*)

original alarm to the switchboard operator and then join the person who discovered the fire and attempt to hold or extinguish it with the fire fighting equipment available.

The telephone operator, if there is an alarm box connected to the city headquarters, shall immediately transmit the box and verify the transmission by calling fire headquarters.

All patients should be removed from involved zones lest their curiosity or anxiety hamper fighting activity or cause themselves injury. The removal of patients may be conducted by rolling or sliding beds or mattresses through horizontal exits or removal by the use of emergency carries. Preparedness to cope with unexpected situations in the care and treatment of the ill, injured, and the aged is vitally important.

A pool of employees should be set up near the switchboard in order to have a uniform supply of personnel who may be needed, and not have to call all over the building for help.

A control center should be established by the security department in the area of the main desk. Such information as floor plans and location of all control valves, switches, first aid and fire fighting equipment, and other pertinent data should be available.

A complete list of names, addresses, and telephone numbers of employees should be kept up to date; emergency telephone numbers of the police, fire, hospital, Red Cross, welfare bureau, doctors, and any other person of authority should also be available here at this control center.

An auxiliary fire alarm system and/or automatic heat or smoke detectors provides an immediate alert to the occupants and utilizes the municipal fire alarm facilities to transmit an alarm to the fire department.

Evacuation: Horizontal

A hospital building constructed of fire resistive material has corridors equipped with fire walls, fire doors, smoke barriers, and totally enclosed vertical openings. The movement of persons can be made by bed, wheel chair, stretcher cart, stretcher, blanket, carries/drags, or a combination of any or all of these methods.

Evacuation: Vertical

Downward movement takes place via enclosed stairwells remote from one another.

The building elevator is not to be depended upon as a method of conveying persons to safe areas, for power failure or other mechanical causes might place them out of service. The elevator should be assigned to the fire department for use in reaching the upper portions of the building.

Patients in wheelchairs, on stretcher carts, and on blankets can be moved via "safe" elevators. The two man swing carry, the four and three man blanket carries should be used for stairwell evacuation.

Successful fire drills should be conducted, without disturbing the patients, by advanced planning in the choice of location of the simulated emergency, and closing the doors to patients' rooms in the vicinity prior to the initiation of the fire drill.

In the event of a fire or other emergency, the smoke barrier doors located in the corridors should be used as the dividing point and should determine the movement of the persons toward stairwells on a horizontal plane. If vertical movement becomes necessary, exit should lead through stairwells free of fire downward to safety.

The housing of patients may be set up on the main (first) floor which is large enough to hold beds, stretcher, carts, cots, etc. if necessary. This would also serve as a first aid station. Ample cots should be available and arrangements should be made with the Red Cross and with the various local hospitals to assist. Each member of the staff should be given a manual of the necessary functions to be performed by them. All charts should be handy at nurses stations to be picked up and used as a means of checking persons moved, (to account for all persons). Guards should be appointed for each entrance door to keep out all unauthorized persons at a time of emergency.

Keys should be available near the switchboard and properly tagged for the laundry, linen supply rooms, storeroom, and drug supplies.

Provision should be made for the transfer of oxygen with the patient, and also to have on hand, at a remote location, a supply which may be needed.

Arrangements should be made with all groups of welfare and other organizations who may render assistance concerning what each organization can supply, how long it will take to fill request, who shall be contacted, and how contact is to be made.

HOSPITAL FIRE SAFETY

Definitions

CONTROL CENTER: There should be established a control

center in close proximity to the telephone operator's room. A security officer should be assigned to this post to issue orders, with an alternate appointed.

DISPATCH CENTER: There should be established a dispatch center in the cafeteria where all employees not directly charged with fire fighting duties or assisting patients will assemble. Employees will be dispatched from this center to areas where assistance is requested, by the officer assigned at this post, with an alternate appointed.

FIRE BRIGADE: A team of employees trained in the various phases of first aid fire fighting is necessary.

INFORMATION CENTER: An information center is to be set up in the main lobby. Security should control movement of elevators and people coming into the hospital from this location.

POINTS OF ASSEMBLY: Lounges or recreation rooms in nurses' residence and intern quarters are to be assembly points. Security is to be in charge and responsible for having someone at the telephone, with alternates appointed.

FIRE DEPARTMENT WATCH: Security officers should be stationed at the front and back entrances of the hospital to direct the fire department to the scene of the fire.

General Rules for All Floors — To Be Posted

If you detect fire or smoke, remember: DO NOT SHOUT FIRE. Be calm — fear and panic can do as much damage as fire. Remove any patients in immediate danger to a safe area.

1. Notify the hospital telephone switchboard operator immediately so that the fire department can be called.
2. Give exact location of fire or smoke. Speak in a moderate tone, so that patients will not overhear and become panic-stricken.
3. Give a brief description of what is burning.
4. Use proper equipment to fight fire. (Every security guard, nurse, and orderly should know the location of fire extin-

guishers in his or her department and understand instructions for operating them.)

5. Close all doors and windows to cut off the oxygen supply.
6. Shut off fans, ventilating systems, and air conditioning units.
7. Shut off gas and electric equipment.
8. Leave all electric lights on.
9. If patients are being moved, one responsible person must check to see that all are removed. If during visiting hours, keep visitors with patients.
10. Turn off at once any oxygen tank in operation.

Duties of Personnel in Case of Fire

SWITCHBOARD OPERATOR

1. Notify the fire department by transmitting the fire alarm, if not automatic.
2. Call the fire department. The fire department number should be posted on the switchboard. Give the exact location of fire or smoke, along with building number and floor.
3. Call the director of the hospital.
4. Call the director of security.
5. Call the assistant director of the hospital.
6. Call the director of nurses.
7. Call the boiler room so that air conditioning systems and ventilating fans can be shut off.
8. Call the nurses residence and request they stand by for instructions.
9. Call the residents and interns quarters and request they stand by for instructions.
10. Remain at the switchboard to give and receive instructions.

BUSINESS OFFICE

1. All employees will report to the chief accountant, who shall be responsible for the money, valuables, records,

books, etc. and shall see that same are removed from the building, if necessary.

2. Shut off all electrical appliances.
3. Post a guard to protect records removed.
4. Report to dispatch center.

KITCHEN

1. Cooks will cover greases or fats on stoves, turn off gas burners and steam cabinets.
2. Maids will turn off gas and disconnect cords of all electrical appliances.
3. Maids will turn off steam and coffee urns.
4. Dishwashers will shut down dishwashing machines.
5. Report to dispatch center.

LINEN ROOM

1. Maids, ward maids, and porters remain on duty.
2. Assemble bathrobes, blankets, etc.
3. Someone of authority will be stationed at the telephone to receive instruction as to what and where to dispatch the necessary articles.

OPERATING ROOM SUPERVISOR

1. Responsible for all general rules.
2. Notify all surgeons of the fire situation and alert them of the possible necessity of the movement of patients. Surgeons in the midst of an operation will determine when their patients are to be moved.
3. Call the dispatch center for any additional help which may be necessary.
4. Move all patients to a safe area beyond the fire door on the same floor.
5. Have sufficient nurses with the patients. Additional help may be obtained from one of the points of assembly.
6. A thorough search must be made to insure the removal of all persons.
7. Inform the fire department of the condition of patients.

NURSERY AND MATERNITY ROOMS

1. Have each mother report to the nursery door, if possible, to pick up her baby.
2. Provide assistance to mothers needing extra care.

3. Guide mothers and babies to a safe area beyond the fire doors on the same floor.
4. Telephone to an assembly point for additional nurses necessary to cope with the situation at hand.
5. Check the records, making a thorough search to insure the removal of all babies and their mothers.

LAUNDRY
1. Close all doors and windows.
2. Shut off fans and ventilating systems.
3. Shut off all electrical appliances, gas equipment.TURN ALL LIGHTS ON.
4. Report to dispatch center.

X-RAY
1. Close all doors, windows, and transoms.
2. Turn off current on all X-ray equipment.

LABORATORY AND PHARMACY
1. Turn off gas and electric appliances.
2. Properly cover or place in closed containers all flammable compounds or materials.
3. Stand by for instructions.
4. If necessary to leave the building, take all important records with you.

ALL CLEAR
When the emergency is over, the chief of the fire department will notify the director, who in turn will notify all nursing stations, control center, dispatch center, information center, and all points of assembly.

Fire Extinguishers

Know your fire extinguishers and how to use them, before fire strikes.

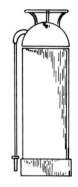

Type: Soda and Acid

Use On: Wood, Paper, Textiles, Rubbish.

Action: Cooling and quenching action.

How to Use: Carry to fire in upright position, grasp nozzle in right hand, raise to the top ring and grasp same. With the left hand grasp the bottom of the extinguisher and invert. Direct the stream at the base of the flames. Get as close as possible. Range of extinguisher is approximately 30 to 40 feet.

Type: Foam

Use On: Oil, Grease, Flammable Liquids.

Action: Smothering or blanketing effect.

How to Use: Carry to fire in upright position, grasp nozzle in right hand, raise to the top ring and grasp same. With the left hand grasp the bottom of the extinguisher and invert. Direct the stream so as to form a blanket over the burning oil or grease. Range of extinguisher is approximately 30 to 40 feet.

Type: Cartridge Operated.

Use On: Wood, Paper, Textiles, Rubbish.

Action: Cooling and quenching action.

How to   Carry to fire in upright position, grasp nozzle in
Use: right hand, with the left hand grasp the bottom
             of extinguisher and invert. When extinguisher is
             turned over and held by the handle provided in
             the base, it must be bumped on the floor to
             puncture the gas cartridge. This releases gas
             from the cartridge and provides pressure for the
             stream. Direct the stream at the base of the
             flames. Get as close as possible. Range of
             extinguisher is approximately 40 to 50 feet.

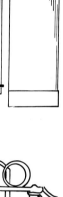

Type: CO_2 (Carbon Dioxide)

Use On: Electrical equipment, confined fires of oil and
             grease.

Action: Extinguishing   action   is   that   primarily   of
             smothering.

How to   Carry to fire, pull lock pin, release horn and
Use: hold by insulated rubber handle on 15 lb. size
             or over. On the smaller sizes 2½ to 5 lb. the
             horn must be raised to a horizontal position.
             Squeeze lever and carrying handle together.
             Move horn across and directly at base of fire.
             Get close. Range of this extinguisher is approxi-
             mately 6 to 8 feet.

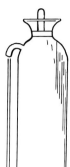

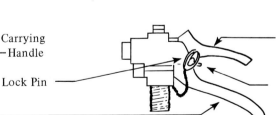

Carrying
Handle   Lever release
                                                To Open: Squeeze
                                                To Close: Release
Lock Pin   Lead & Wire Seal

ENLARGED VIEW OF HANDLE

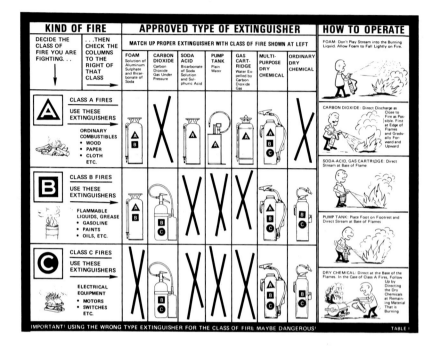

Figure 32. (*Courtesy of* National Institute for Occupational Safety and Health.)

APPENDIX

Fire Report

DRILL_____

FALSE ALARM_____

FIRE_____

LOCATION_____ DATE _____

TIME STARTED_____ TIME OF ALARM _____

BY TELEPHONE_____ BY PULL STATION _____

Time first response by brigade_____

Total responding personnel_____

Was hospital fire truck or other equipment brought to scene   YES_____

NO_____

GENERAL REMARKS (Fire Marshall or reporting authority)

_____

_____

_____

_____

_____

COMMENTS BY OBSERVERS

_____

_____

_____

_____

Courtesy of Saint Joseph's Hospital and Medical Center, Paterson, New Jersey.

Special Fire Report

Date of fire: _____Time of fire:_____ ( ) AM
( ) PM

Building: _____Location: _____

Alarm box: _____Type of fire: _____

Fire reported by:_____Dept. _____

Alarm turned in: ( ) yes ( ) no   If no please give reason below:

_____

Equipment used: _____

_____

Cause of fire: _____

_____

_____

NOTATION: _____

_____

_____

Area Declared Safe By: _____

Patrolman:_____Badge # _____

FOLLOW UP REPORT:

Officer Reporting:_____ Date: _____

Equipment Replaced:_____ Date: _____

Notations: _____

_____

_____

Signature:_____Badge #_____

Courtesy of Holy Name Hospital, Teaneck, New Jersey.

Fire Drill Report

Date:

Date of drill:_____Time of drill:_____Time of all clear: _____

Alarm box:_____Code: _____

Alarm turned in by:_____Title:_____

Person(s) supervising drill:

Name:_____Title:_____Area:_____

_____   _____   _____

_____   _____   _____

_____   _____   _____

_____   _____   _____

_____   _____   _____

Security officer on duty: _____Title:_____

_____Title:_____

_____Title:_____

Patrolman on duty: _____Post: _____

_____Post: _____

_____Post: _____

_____Post: _____

Main alarm box reset by: _____

Nursing supervisor:_____

Notation:

Signature: _____

Fire Equipment Report

TO: Plant Engineer

FROM: Director of Security

SUBJECT: Request for Repair or Installation of Fire Fighting and/or Fire Safety
             Equipment

REQUISTION FOR: ( ) INSTALLATION OF NEW EQUIPMENT

                    ( ) REPAIR OF EXISTING EQUIPMENT

LOCATION: _____

REASON FOR REQUEST: *(Explain problem or need for equipment)*

_____

_____

_____

_____   _____
Signature of Reporting Officer   Signature of Director of Security

----

Disposition of Request

TO: Director of Security

FROM: Plant Engineer

SUBJECT: Fire Equipment Requisition

Equipment Installed or Repaired?   Please Specify.

_____

No Action Taken — Reason: _____

_____

                              _____
                              Signature of Plant Engineer

SELECTED READINGS

Aetna Casualty and Security Co.: *Make Our Hospitals Fire Safe*. Cat. #300284, 1965.

Babcock, Chester I.: Nursing Hose Life Safety: A trend for the better. *Fire Jounal*, January 1967.

Boissoneau, Robert A.: Continuing fire protection education for hospital personnel, *Fire Jounal*, May 1968.

———: The occupancy fire picture continuing fire protection education for hospital personnel. *Fire Journal*, May 1968.

Bravos, T. A.: Why not integrate fire and police services. *Mental Hospitals*, II, 55-56, June 1960.

Bryan, John L.: Developing employee fire consciousness. *Industrial Security*, April 1959.

Burgun, J. Armand: Life safety code protects lives not just buildings. *Hospitals*, J.A.H.S., January 1, 1968.

Cihlar, Carroll: Ohio nursing home fire: an analysis. *Hospitals*, J.A.H.A., 44: March 1, 1970.

Crowe J. M.: Effective training reduces fire losses. *Industrial Security*, 4 (No. 2): 10-12, April 1960.

Extinguishers described for three fire classes. *Hospitals*, J.A.H.A., January 16, 1967.

Fire hazards in oxygen enriched atmospheres. *Hospitals*, J.A.H.A., February 1, 1967.

Grimshaw, Joseph N.: Fires are up Our guard is down. *Hospital Management*, July 1967.

Harris, A. Everett, Jr.: Smoke I a hazard in hospital fires. *Safety Newsletter*, Hospital Section, National Safety Council, June 1970.

Hayt, Emanuel: No proof negligence of hospital caused fire in patient's bed. *LL.B. Hospital Management*, January 1967.

Hospital Emergency Preparedness, NFPA No. 3m. 1970.

Hospital Fire Safety Program. Jersey City, The Jersey City Fire Department and The Jersey City Medical Center.

Industrial Fire Brigades Training Manual. NFPA, 1968.

Jacobs, Eleanor A. and Reith, Bernard G.: Testing flame-retardant linen for hospital use. *Hospital*, J.A.H.A., May 16, 1968.

Karshmer, Norman M. and Lubin, David: Smoke makes fire drills more effective. *Modern Hospital*, May 1967.

La Bush, Isadore and Goldin, Sidney: An award-winning program for fire safety training. *Hospitals*, J.A.H.A., July 16, 1967.

Maddox, Darrell: Detection system and design protect hospital against fire. *Modern Hospitals*, August 1969.

McCormick, James M., M.D.: NFPA standards for hospitals. *Fire Journal*, November, 1969.

Meyer, Edward J.: Design for a hospital fire safety program. *Security World, 1* (No. 1): July 1964.

National Fire Protection Association: *Guard Operations in Fire Lost Prevention.* Boston, NFPA, 1968.

Nursing home fire defense. *Nursing Home Administrator, 20* #3: May-June 1966.

Palmer, Robert T.: Emergency planning for hospitals. *Fire Journal, 63* No. 2, March 1969.

Security Guidelines For Hospitals. The Greater New York Hospital Association, New York, 1968.

Shaw, A. J.: How to handle flammables in your hospital. *Modern Hospital,* December 1968.

Stevens, Richard E.: Designing life safety in institutional occupancies. *Fire Journal,* May 1967.

Stimson, Donald L.: Designing a fire detection system for a large hospital. *Fire Journal,* March 1973.

Unique extinguishing system protects computers. *Bldg. Maintenance and Modernization,* October 1968.

Chapter 19

BOMB THREATS AND
HOW TO HANDLE THEM

E VERY hospital is subject to the possible threat of a bomb scare. Most bomb threats are made by psychotics, pranksters, and extremists. A bomb threat at a hospital, however, cannot be taken lightly. A detailed plan of action for meeting a bomb threat should be developed.

When drafting a "bomb threat plan," it is a good policy for the security department to consult with the chief hospital administrator and his staff, nursing and custodial divisions, local police and fire departments, and neighboring hospital systems that have instituted such plans. The final plan should be disseminated at least to all administrative personnel.

The following general procedures should be observed when a bomb threat report is received by a hospital.

1. *The person receiving the call is to try to get as much information as possible from the person calling.* Many factors can be determined about the person calling just by hearing the person speak, such as approximate age, local accent, or a distinctive accent. These clues would be very helpful to the investigator when he arrives. The main thing for the person receiving the threat is *not to panic.*

Write down everything possible as to what the caller said and how he said it. If possible, try to keep the caller talking. Find out where the bomb is placed, the time it is expected to go off, the type of bomb, etc. (See "Bomb Threat Checklist" in chapter Appendix.)

2. *Notify the chief hospital administrator and the security director.*

3. *Telephone the police department.* The senior security officer on duty should immediately report the bomb threat to the police department and request police assistance at the hospital.

4. *Conduct a search.* Place into action predesignated search teams. When looking for the bomb always remember that the most effective search is done by people working in the building, i.e. security personnel, housekeeping personnel, and head nurses. They know their immediate work area and can easily spot something that does not belong there. A security officer should be put in charge to organize the search until the appropriate law enforcement personnel arrive. A command post should be established at a central location.

5. *Strange objects (possible explosives) are not to be handled.* Bombs may be hidden in anything, such as lunch boxes, thermos bottles, attache cases, and paper bags. The search team should look for something that does not belong where it is. When you find something that you think may be a bomb, *do not touch it.* The area should be closed off and the object that may turn out to be explosive should be handled only by experienced officials, such as the local police department, the fire department, military, or other bomb disposal experts.

6. *Evacuate the area.* When a suspected explosive object is found, the security officer should report his findings to the chief hospital administrator and/or his delegate. The police and fire department should be thoroughly informed of the suspected object's discovery and its exact location. The security officer now should keep everyone clear of the object, turn off all office machines, air conditioners, etc., open all doors and windows in the area, and direct the disposal team to the object when they arrive. The lights should be kept on to assist the disposal team. If the object should explode, the open windows and doors will allow the blast to vent and thus reduce the damaging affects.

If a suspected object is found in or near patient's rooms, the security officer should move the patients and personnel located alongside and directly above and below to a reasonably safe location. If it becomes necessary to evacuate the entire hospital, or any major part thereof, it is up to the hospital administrator and/or his delegate to issue the orders.

A hospital does not easily lend itself to total evacuation. Even partial evacuation with ambulatory patients is a serious problem.

The established fire drill procedures should be used in either the partial or total evacuation of the premises.

Additional General Factors to Consider

1. Remain cool and calm at all times.
2. Make proper notifications and assignments promptly.
3. Do not create a panic amongst the patients and staff.
4. Cooperate with police and fire officials.
5. Try to remember all facts for a complete report.

A Checklist for Bomb Threats

Most often, bomb threats are received over the telephone and usually to the first person that answers. For this reason, switchboard operators, secretaries, security personnel, and the nursing staff should have specific directives for obtaining as much information as they can from the caller. Familiarity with the checklist for bomb threats in the chapter appendix could assist the authorities in locating the bomb and/or the caller.

APPENDIX

Bomb Threat Checklist

Caller's Identity: Name_____

Male_____Female_____

Approximate Age_____

Caller's Origin: Internal____Long Distance____Local____Other____

Caller's Message: (Write it down exactly as given — Do not interrupt caller)

Questions to ask the caller:

1. What time is the explosive set to go off?_____AM/PM

2. The exact location of the explosive? _____

_____

3. The type of explosive: TNT____dynamite____powder____other____

Caller's Distinguishing Traits:

Voice Pitch	*Speech*	**Accent*	*Language*	*Manner*	*Background Noises*
Low__	Slow__	Foreign__	Poor__	Angry__	Traffic__
Loud__	Fast__	American__	Fair__	Calm__	Construction__
Deep__	Stutter__	*Explain	Good__	Rational__	Music__
High__	Precise__	_____	Excellent__	Irrational__	Quiet__
Nasal__	Muffled__		Dirty__	Emotional__	Party Noises__
Hoarse__	Other__			Deliberate__	Office Mach.__
Other__				Laughing__	Factory Mach.__
				Other__	Animals__
					Other__

SELECTED READINGS

Berlow, Leonard: What to do when you get a bomb threat. *Modern Hospital,* December 1968.

Bombs and Explosives. Lafayette, Purdue University.

Brodie, Thomas G.: *Bombs and Bombings.* Springfield, Thomas, 1973.

Donovan, Robert: A manual for bomb attacks. *Security World,* 5 (No. 5): May 1968.

Guidelines for dealing with bomb threats. *National Association of Secondary School Principals, #96:* January-February 1971.

Lenz, Robert R.: *Explosives and Bomb Disposal Guide.* Springfield, Thomas, 1973.

McGuire, E. Patrick: When bombing threatens. *The Conference Board Record, VII, #9:* 57-63, September 1971.

Pike, Earl A.: *Protection Against Bombs and Incendiaries.* Springfield, Thomas, 1973.

Plant protection — a bomb is the problem. *Business Week,* March 21, 1951.

Pointer, Homer F.: Bomb threats to public schools. *Industrial Security,* June, 1966.

Ronayne, John A.: Bomb Threats In Industrial Plant. *Industrial Security,* October 1959.

Security Guidelines For Hospitals. New York, The Greater New York Hospital Association, 1968.

Staffel, Major Joseph: *Explosives and Homemade Bombs.* Springfield, Thomas, 1972.

Chapter 20

HOSPITAL SAFETY

THE security force of any organization becomes the eyes and ears for the administrative staff. As a guard makes rounds, he should be constantly alert to unsafe conditions that may cause an injury. All unsafe conditions should be immediately reported to the proper authorities.

At least 95 percent of all accidents are caused by an unsafe practice or an unsafe condition. Unsafe practices are any action which increases the risk of an accident by an employee. Unsafe conditions are faulty or negligent hazards which increase the risk of an accident.

Unsafe Practices

1. Failure to warn coworkers of possible hazards.
2. Positioning oneself in an unsafe area.
3. Horseplay.
4. Lifting with ones back and not with legs.
5. Removing safety guards or devices.
6. Operating or working at unsafe speeds.
7. Not wearing personal protective equipment.
8. Smoking in prohibited areas.
9. Disregard of safety rules and signs.
10. Taking unnecessary risks.

Unsafe Conditions

1. Absence of adequate warning systems.
2. Defective fire fighting equipment.
3. Inadequate lighting.
4. Protruding objects.
5. Unsafe electrical system.
6. Poor evacuation system.

7. Absence of proper safety guards.
8. Poor ventilation.
9. Poor fire and explosion protection.
10. Poor general physical conditions.

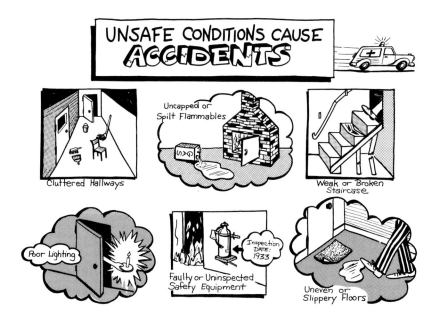

Figure 33. (*Courtesy of* Rutgers University Curriculum Laboratory.)

There are seven basic actions to look for when observing for hazards.

1. Falling.
2. Overexertion.
3. Getting caught on.
4. Getting struck against.
5. Getting caught between.
6. Getting struck by.
7. Illness.

Hospital security officers have four main areas of safety concern: Safety for oneself, for hospital employees, for hospital patients, and for hospital visitors.

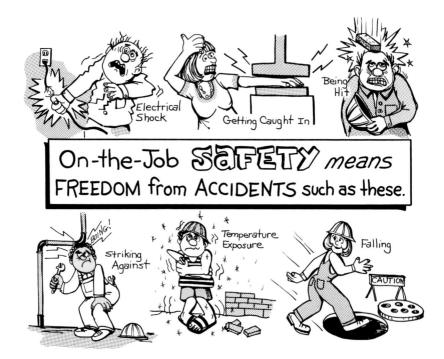

Figure 34. (*Courtesy of* Rutgers University Curriculum Laboratory.)

Every hospital security officer should follow the following practices.

- Think, act, and practice safety.
- Report all unsafe conditions so that corrective action can be taken.
- Avoid playing practical jokes or engaging in horseplay.
- Observe all safety rules and regulations.
- Know the hospital's fire safety evacuation plan (see chapter 18).
- Know what to do in the event of fire or other emergencies.
- Know the proper procedures for lifting with legs, not back.
- Enforce no smoking regulations especially in areas that have oxygen or other highly flammable materials in use.
- Constantly remain alert. Carelessness leads to accidents.

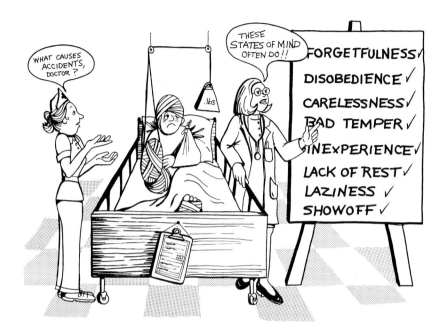

Figure 35. (*Courtesy of* Rutgers University Curriculum Laboratory.)

Hazard Spotter Checklist*

The following list of hazards is intended to serve as a check-list on unsafe acts and unsafe conditions in every hospital department and in every type of work situation. Keep these hazards in mind as you make your daily tour of the hospital.

Improper Safety Attitude

—"Can't happen to me" attitude.
—Excuses such as "I didn't know it was a safety rule — no one told me."

---

*Reprinted, with permission, from *Safety Guide for Health Care Institutions,* a joint publication of the American Hospital Association and the National Safety Council.

Clothing and Protective Equipment

___Loose, excessively soiled, ill-fitting, or inadequate clothing.

___Incorrect type of protective equipment; incorrect adjustment.

___Absence of needed gloves, aprons, safety shoes, or eye protections.

___Dangerous use of rings or other jewelry around machinery.

Work Area

___Poor housekeeping.

___Inadequate or glaring illumination.

___Excessive noise.

___Inadequate ventilation.

___Temperature extremes (too hot or too cold).

___Cramped quarters; hazards from nearby operations.

___Exposure to dust, fumes, gases.

___Lack of signs or warning devices.

___Footing: uneven, slippery, obstructed, unstable.

___Insecure overhead material.

___Insecure piling or storage; excessive loading.

Faulty Job Preparation

___Failure to provide illumination and ventilation.

___Failure to secure, fasten, align, or prepare material.

___Failure to remove hot substances or cool off equipment before starting work.

___Failure to obtain help or mechanical handling equipment for lifting and carrying.

___Failure to remove tools and other objects near running machinery.

Faulty Job Performance

___Failure to de-energize or ground electrical circuits.

___Handling of repairs or adjustments without a qualified repairman or electrician.

—Unsafe loading, unloading, piling.
—Rough handling of equipment, material.
—Working at unsafe speed.
—Failure to face ladder.
—Working too close together.
—Getting on or off machinery or equipment when it is in operation.
—Working on or near moving parts.
—Horseplay.
—Looking at welding arc without protection.

Improper Operation of Equipment

—Unauthorized use of equipment.
—Failure to signal, warn, post warning signs.
—Failure to lock out, shut off, and tag electrical switch.
—Failure to secure vehicles and materials from sliding or moving.

Neglect or Improper Use of Safety Devices

—Failure to use, remove, or disconnect equipment, hoses, wires.
—Rendering equipment inoperative; plugging outlets, damaging electrical plugs.
—Improper use of safety equipment; improper adjustment.
—Replacement with an unsafe device.

Unsafe Use of Proper Equipment

—Defectiveness of proper equipment; use of it beyond its capacity.
—Wrong positioning of equipment.
—Improper fastening, adjustment.
—Unsafe speed.

Use of Wrong Equipment

—Use of wrong tool or device, wrong type or size.

__Makeshift, improvised equipment; use of hands and shoes instead of tools or devices.
__Use of flammables or explosives instead of safe solvents.
__Causing chips by striking tools or objects of the same hardness.

Unsafe Movement, Posture

__Wrong lifting; lack of balance.
__Incorrect or insecure grip.
__Running, jumping.
__Striking against object while straightening up or bending over.

Unsafe Positions

__Standing over or in front of apparatus instead of to one side.
__Overreaching.
__Insecure or slippery support.
__Walking over, instead of around.
__Wrong riding of vehicles, loads.
__Standing under working crews or under loads that are suspended or likely to fall.
__Standing too close to moving machinery.
__Failure to allow for pinch points.
__Walking on wrong side of corridor or roadway.
__Unwarranted use of shortcuts.

Machinery

__Lack of guarding; inadequate or weak guarding.
__Unsafe starting or stopping devices.
__Lack of positive electrical lockout protection.
__Unguarded flying material.
__Lack of signs; obscured or improper location of signs.

Material Handling

__Materials or objects: heavy, unwieldy, rough, sharp, hot, corrosive.

—Unsafe handling equipment: containers, carts, trucks, ambulances, other vehicles, conveyors, hoists.

Tools

—Wrong tool for the job.
—Unsafe condition.
—Use in unsafe position.
—Placement in unsafe position.
—Lack of electrical safety in use of appliances.
—Improper guarding for power-actuated devices.

Delayed First Aid

—Failure to report accidents.
—Delay in reporting accidents.
—Self-administered "treatment."

SELECTED READINGS

American Insurance Association, Engineering and Safety Department: *Your Guide to Safety As a Hospital Employee.* 1961.

Annual Administrative Reviews Safety. *Hospitals,* J.A.H.A., March 1, 1966.

Bakko, Orville E.: Employee safety program. *Hospitals,* J.A.H.A., 44: June 1970.

Bowles, Grower C., Jr.: Safe ventilation and storage are essential in pharmacy. *Modern Hospitals,* November 1969.

Brow, Miner L.: Safety . . . An individual responsibility. *National Safety News,* August 1970.

Burgun, Armand: Life safety code protects lives, not just buildings. *Hospitals,* J.A.H.A., June 1969.

Conductive flooring principles are easily explained. *Hospitals,* J.A.H.A., October 16, 1967.

Day, Savannah S. and Hodges, Marianne B.: Factors affecting skid resistance of hard floor surfaces. *Hospital* J.A.H.A., April 16, 1967.

Electrical Plugs and Reciptacles Standardized for Safety. *Hospitals,* J.A.H.A., July 16, 1968.

Engineering and maintenance digest essentials of ladder safety. *Hospitals,* J.A.H.A., November 1, 1967.

Giant matchbook gives patients safety tips. *Hospitals*, J.A.H.A., June 16, 1967.

Holthouser, Ralph H., Jr.: Safety in central service. *Hospital Management*, June 1967.

Hospitals: Manufacturers need greater awareness of electrical hazards. *Hospitals*, J.A.H.A., November 16, 1968.

Hospital Occupational Health Services Study, Employee Health and Safety Statistics and Records, Vol. II, U.S. Department of Health, Education, and Welfare, March 1975.

Katz, Eli G.: Evaluation of hospital essential electrical systems. *Fire Journal*, November 1968.

Lubin, David: Electrical safety. *Hospitals*, J.A.H.A., December 1, 1969.

Lubin, David, Hinkes, Jules M., and Karshmer, Norman M.: How to Insure Safety In Electrically Operated Beds.

Nader, Ralph: In hospital and industry we must insist on safety. *Modern Hospital*, February 1968.

Pedersen, Thomas: Accident exposure in mental hospitals. *Safety Newsletter*, Hospital Section National Safety Council, July 1970.

Plants help eliminate traffic problems. *Hospitals*, J.A.H.A., September 16, 1969.

Role of the security department in safety. *Security Education Briefs*, (OAK Security Inc.), 2, No. 11:

Safety Guide for Health Care Institutions. Chicago, American Hospital Association and The National Safety Council, 1972.

Schneider, William J.: Poor records can block improvements in safety. *Hospitals*, J.A.H.A., June 16, 1967.

The hospitals liability for injuries on its premises. *Hospitals*, J.A.H.A., July 1, 1966.

The problem employee. *National Safety News*, 101, No. 1: January 1970.

Thompson, Robert E.: Electrostatic safety in clothing. *Fire Journal*, November 1969.

Waite, Richard: Hospital safety needed. *Journal of Environmental Health*, November/December 1969.

Walter, Carl, M.D.: Safe electric environment in the hospital. *Bulletin American College of Surgeons*, 54, No. 4, July-August, 1969.

Walter, Carl, M.D.: New concept: Safe patient power center. *Modern Hospitals*, June 1969.

What hospitals are doing to cut down accidents. *U.S. News and World Report*, March 29, 1976.

Chapter 21

THE OCCUPATIONAL SAFETY AND HEALTH ACT OF 1970

THE Occupational Safety and Health Act of 1970, OSHA, became an official part of national labor law on April 28, 1971. The mission as declared by Congress is "to assure so far as possible every working man and woman in the Nation safe and healthful working conditions and to preserve our human resources . . ."

Congress was specific on how OSHA was to be implemented:

- by encouraging employers and employees to reduce hazards in the work place, and start or improve existing safety and health programs,
- by establishing employer and employee responsibilities;
- by authorizing OSHA to set mandatory job safety and health standards;
- by providing an effective enforcement program;
- by encouraging the states to assume the fullest responsibility for administering and enforcing their own occupational safety and health programs that are to be at least as effective as the federal program;
- by providing for reporting procedures on job inquiries, illnesses, and fatalities.

Coverage by the Act

The Act covers every employer in a business affecting commerce who has one or more employees. The Act does not affect workplaces covered under other federal laws, such as the Coal Mine Health and Safety Act and the Federal Metal and Nonmetallic Safety Act.

Federal, state, and local government employees are covered under separate provisions in the Act for public employment.

167

Standards

OSHA adopts standards and, among other methods for accomplishing compliance, conducts inspections of workplaces to determine whether the standards are being met. A safety or health standard is a legally enforceable regulation governing conditions, practices, or operations to assure safe and healthful workplaces.

A compliance officer looks for compliance with national safety and health standards when he inspects a workplace. He is concerned with what standards apply there and whether the employer and employees are complying with them.

The standards are published in the Federal Register. All amendments, corrections, insertions, or deletions involving standards also are printed in the Federal Register.

The Role of Employers

The Act requires each employer to provide a workplace free from safety and health hazards and to comply with the standards.

Employer Responsibilities

- be aware that you have a general duty responsibility to provide a place of employment free from recognized hazards and to comply with occupational safety and health standards promulgated under the Act;
- familiarize yourself with mandatory occupational safety and health standards;
- make sure your employees know about OSHA;
- examine conditions in your workplace to make sure they conform to applicable safety and health standards;
- remove or guard hazards;
- make sure your employees have and use safe tools and equipment, including required personal protective gear, and that they are properly maintained;

- use color codes, posters, labels, or signs to warn employees of potential hazards;
- establish or update operating procedures and communicate them so that employees follow safety and health requirements for their own protection;
- provide medical examinations when required by OSHA standards;
- keep required OSHA records of work-related injuries and illnesses (if you have eight or more employees), and post the annual summary during the entire month of February each year;
- report, to the nearest OSHA area office, each injury or health hazard that results in a fatality or hospitalization of five or more employees;
- post, in the workplace, the OSHA poster informing employees of their rights and responsibilities;
- advise OSHA compliance officers of authorized employee representatives to permit their participation in the inspection walkaround. If there are no such representatives, allow a reasonable number of employees to confer with the compliance officer during the walkaround;
- do NOT discriminate against employees who properly exercise their rights under the Act;
- post OSHA citations of violations of standards at the worksite involved;
- seek advice and consultation as needed by writing, calling, or visiting the nearest OSHA office (OSHA will not inspect you just because you call for assistance);
- be active in your (hospital) association's involvement in job safety and health.

The Role of Employees

The Act requires each employee to comply with occupational safety and health standards, as well as all rules, regulations, and orders issued under the Act that apply to his or her own actions and conduct.

Employee Responsibilities

- read the OSHA poster at your jobsite;
- comply with any applicable OSHA standards;
- follow all of your employer's safety and health standards and rules;
- wear or use prescribed protective equipment;
- report hazardous conditions to your supervisor;
- report any job-related injuries or illnesses to your employer and seek treatment promptly;
- cooperate with the OSHA compliance officer conducting an inspection if he inquires about conditions at your jobsite;
- use your rights under the Act responsibly.

Penalties

The Act provides for mandatory penalties against employers of up to $1,000 for each serious violation and for optional penalties of up to $1,000 for each nonserious violation. Penalties of up to $1,000 per day may be proposed for failure to correct violations within the proposed time period. Also, any employer who willfully or repeatedly violates the Act may be assessed penalties of up to $10,000 for each such violation.

Criminal penalties are also provided for in the Act. Any willful violation resulting in death of an employee, upon conviction, is punishable by a fine of not more than $10,000 or by imprisonment for not more than six months or by both. Conviction of an employer after a first conviction doubles these maximum penalties.

Voluntary Activity

While providing penalties for violations, the Act also encourages efforts by labor and management, before an OSHA inspection, to reduce injuries and illnesses arising out of employment.

The Department of Labor encourages employers and employees to reduce workplace hazards voluntarily and to develop and improve safety and health programs in all workplaces and industries.

Such cooperative action would initially focus on the identification and elimination of hazards that could cause death, injury, or illness to employees and supervisors. There are many public and private organizations that can provide information and assistance in this effort, if requested.

Records That Must Be Kept

OSHA requires employers of eight or more employees to keep certain records of job-related fatalities, injuries, and illnesses. OSHA requires that three simple forms must be maintained:

1. OSHA 100 — a log in which each reportable case is entered on a single line.
2. OSHA 101 — a supplementary record with details on each individual case.
3. OSHA 102 — an annual summary compiled from the log. (This summary must be posted in the workplace by February 1 each year and be kept there one month for employee examination).

If there are no recordable deaths, injuries, or illnesses, there is nothing to fill in.

All employers not exempt (those with eight or more employees) from the recordkeeping requirements must have the forms available when an OSHA compliance officer makes an inspection. The forms do not have to be mailed to any OSHA office.

Chapter 22

ORGANIZING A SAFETY COMMITTEE

A SAFETY and health committee, when properly run, can be used to fight more than one battle for management. Once employees are thinking about the workplace from management's point of view — and if management listens to employees — employees will think of some excellent suggestions, ranging from safety and health improvements to time saving to process improvement.

The cost of insurance premiums and of workers' compensation insurance may be lowered as a consequence of committee work. Many employers have reaped substantial savings after an energetic committee brought about a drastic reduction in accidents and injuries.

Genuine support for a working safety committee also presents an opportunity to demonstrate good faith when the OSHA compliance officer comes to the hospital.

Size of the Committee

What kind of committee is needed? How many members should be on it? These are among the first questions that come up when management decides to tackle hospital hazards through an active safety and health committee. The answer most frequently given by experts: Let the size of the hospital and its hazard potential dictate the type and size of the committee.

Most hospitals may prefer to use one central safety and health committee. They should regularly inspect every operation within the hospital complex, exerting an all-out effort to make the hospital completely safe.

Large hospitals may find it necessary to form several active subcommittees that feed into a central committee.

How to Organize the Committee

To command respect, the committee leader or chairman should be a person whose authority exceeds the authority of each member of the group. This gives a fair guarantee of (a) effective, controlled action to follow committee findings and (b) access to the next higher level of management via the committee chairman. Following this general rule, the network of safety and health committees can be set.

- A hospital executive, for example, might be in charge of a committee of department heads.
- Each department head can chair a committee in his section of the hospital.
- A supervisor is the ideal leader for a committee of workers.

What the Safety and Health Committee Does

To be successful, a safety and health committee should be involved in the actual planning of the safety and health program and should have a part in making the program operate. Definite policies should be established at the time the committee is organized. They should include some or all of the following:

- Establish procedures for handling suggestions and recommendations of the committee.
- Inspect a selected area of the establishment each month for the purpose of detecting hazards.
- Conduct regularly scheduled meetings to discuss accident and illness prevention methods, safety and health promotion, hazards noted on inspections, injury and illness records, and other pertinent subjects.
- Investigate accidents and near-accidents as a basis for recommending means to prevent recurrence.
- Provide information on safe and healthful working practices to the hospital administration.
- Recommend changes or additions to improve protective clothing and equipment.

•Develop or revise rules to comply with current safety and health standards.

•Promote safety training for committee members and other employees.

•Promote safety and health programs for all employees.

How to Make a Committee Work

In helping the committee do its most effective work, keep in mind these general guidelines:

•Keep the safety and health committee small so that every member can participate actively.

•If a large hospital has many key people who should function on the central committee, rotate them or invite them as guests at certain meetings.

•The central committee can determine what auxiliary committees are needed in the hospital, and appoint heads of committees on the next lower level; the latter can select their own members to do what needs to be done.

If a job looks too big for a small group, subdivide it, allocating portions of the task to small committees. Everyone on the committee ought to be serving it conspicuously; if not, they are excess baggage.

•Remember that the committee members are not born knowing what it is all about. They have to be taught.

•Management should provide the committee with its direction, its goal, its limits.

•To keep members interested, the committee should meet at least once a month and carry out assignments between meetings, encouraging meaningful research and observation of hospital safety and health hazards.

•In advance of each meeting, the secretary should get a notice to each member. A good practice is to combine this with delivery of a copy of the minutes of the last meeting. It is also the secretary's job to draw up an agenda and clear it with the chairman, who is to conduct the meeting in the order agreed upon.

•Meetings should not last more than one hour. In order to accomplish brief meetings, the secretary should prepare a tight agenda — and this takes time.

•A good meeting program should be established: first, a call to order by the chairman; next, revision of minutes from the previous meeting, followed by a signing of the attendance sheet and reports on past assignments. Suggestions and discussion of work that needs to be done comes next. At all times, the members should be stimulated to come forward with ideas and suggestions. If a member has nothing to contribute, either he is shirking or you do not need him in the group. Before the meeting is adjourned, specific duties should be assigned and accepted, with deadline dates for completion noted in the minutes.

Diplomacy to Achieve Common Goals

It has been a common pitfall for committees to stray from their specific territory. It takes diplomacy to keep spirited discussions on course. There must be a firm rule that no issues other than those concerning safety or health may be brought up at meetings.

At times it is the chairman who must be kept on course. It is easy to slip out of the leader's role as coordinator and try to do the legwork of members. When committee officials step out of character they frustrate the members. If the chairman of the committee does it all himself, the meeting is no longer a committee — it is simply a meeting to hear one man's opinions.

The members should be given the opportunity to participate and also to see that their work is appreciated. Many hospitals have a system of sending copies of minutes to officers and key people throughout the hospital, to keep them posted on the efforts and achievements of the committee.

Avoid Showpiece Committees

Beware of committee lacking authority. The best advice to members of a committee lacking management support is to disband. Committees with no real power degenerate into self-perpetuating institutions with all of the attendant abuses. Those lame-duck committees tend to talk about problems rather than solve them.

Do not let the committee become a vehicle for avoiding responsibility. This is a major claim of weakness held against committees.

Do not let a handful of employees perpetuate themselves in committee duty. Rotate the committee membership; this is the key to a successful committee. Plan a careful system of rotation. Tap the knowledge of experienced workers. One common way — the way the OSHA Advisory Committee works — is through overlapping terms so that there is always a certain percentage of experienced members around.

If you prefer to bring in a whole new group of people each time you rotate the committee, make sure that this new group has adequate technical assistance or includes members with experience in safety and health procedures.

The sooner the new members are given the responsibility to inspect specific areas of the hospital complex, the faster they develop the skills to rout out hazards.

Remember, the most important ingredient is management's commitment. Nothing is more worthless than a showpiece safety and health committee.

INDEX